Exercises in Radiological Diagnosis

W0106469

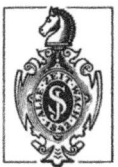

P. Haehnel   Ch. Kleitz

Mammography

83 Radiological Exercises for Students
and Practitioners

In Collaboration with Bernadette Lux

With 142 Illustrations

Springer-Verlag
Berlin Heidelberg New York
London Paris Tokyo

Dr. Pierre Haehnel

Dr. Christian Kleitz

Cabinet de Sénologie

18, rue du 22 Novembre

F-67000 Strasbourg

Translated from the French by

Marie-Thérèse Wackenheim

Library of Congress Cataloging-in-Publication Data. Haehnel, P. (Pierre), 1941- [Mammagraphie. English] Mammography : 83 radiological exercises for students and practitioners / P. Haehnel, Ch. Kleitz ; in collaboration with Bernadette Lux: ; [translated from the French by Marie-Therese Wackenheim]. p. cm.–(Exercises in radiological diagnosis) Translation of: Mammagraphie. Includes index.
ISBN-13: 978-3-540-15328-3   e-ISBN-13: 978-3-642-70383-6
DOI: 10.1007/978-3-642-70383-6
1. Breast–Radiography–Problems, exercises, etc. 2. Breast–Diseases–Diagnosis–Atlases.
I. Kleitz, Ch. (Christian), 1944-   . II. Title. III. Series.
RG493.5.R33H3413 1988   618.1'907572–dc19   88-12350

© Springer-Verlag Berlin Heidelberg 1988

2127/3130-543210 – Printed on acid-free paper

Foreword

When he became Chairman of Radiology in 1959, my predecessor, Professor Ch. M. Gros, founded the Strasbourg School of Senology. Dr. Pierre Haehnel is now the standard-bearer of this very flourishing school. For many years he has been applying himself to maintaining and developing the field of senology in the Faculty of Radiology at Strasbourg, organizing the teaching of this transdisciplinary subject.

Dr. Pierre Haehnel is thus particularly well qualified to write this new book of Exercises in Radiological Diagnosis.

A. WACKENHEIM

Contents

I. Normal Breast

1

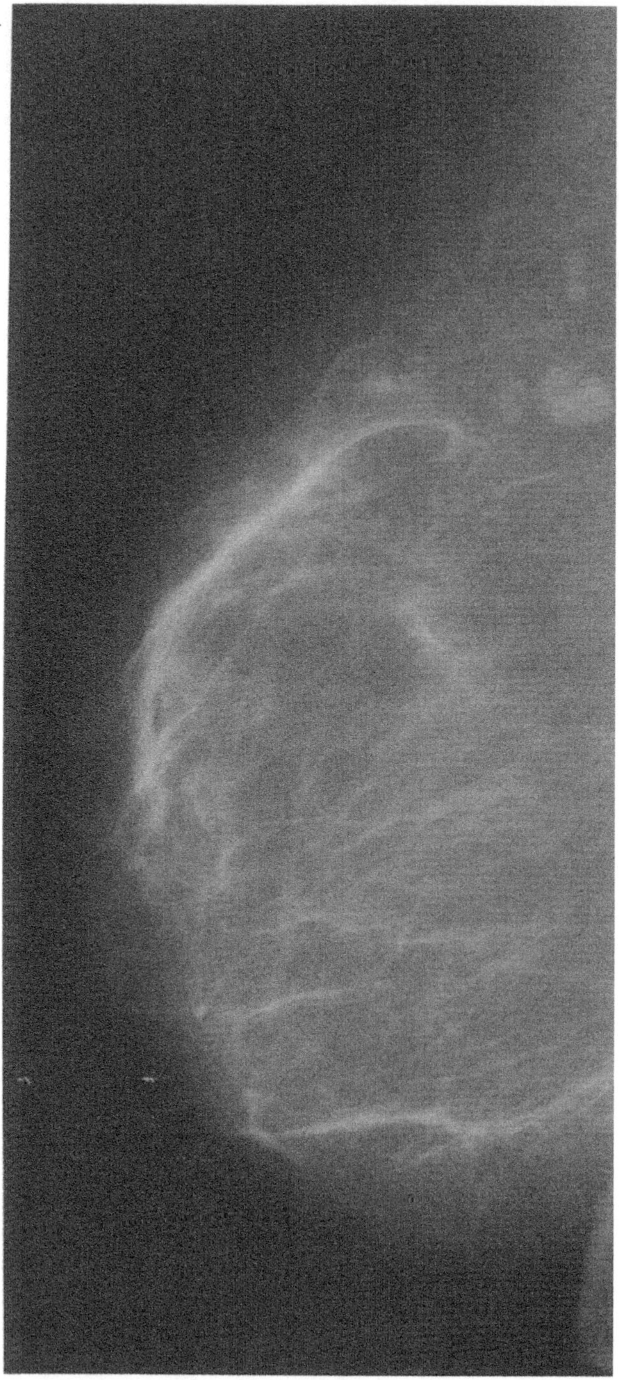

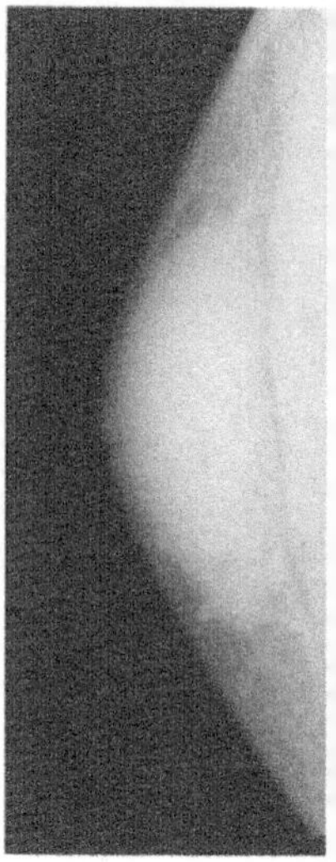

2

Normal breast (lateral view). Radiograph shows the elements of the breast, **1**
namely:
- The well-developed *fatty tissue* which in fact constitutes a natural contrast
  medium
- The supporting *connective tissue,* which is seen as linear and curvilinear
  opacities without any architectural rupture
- The *vascular networks,* visible in the retromammillary area, 4 cm from the
  nipple, as linear opacities with parallel margins, slightly less dense than the
  supporting tissue
- The *nipple* is not visible on tangential views. Note the presence of dense,
  homogeneous, oval opacities in the upper part of t he breast which correspond
  to the normal axillary nodes

Mammary bud. The mammary bud is the first stage in the development of the **2**
mammary gland. It consists of a small retromammillary bud, later hollowed by
the lactiferous ducts.

On radiographs it most often appears, as in the case shown, dense and oval. It
may sometimes have a trident dendritic form, analogous to what is seen in
gynecomastia. Here, the density of the bud is marked and homogeneous.

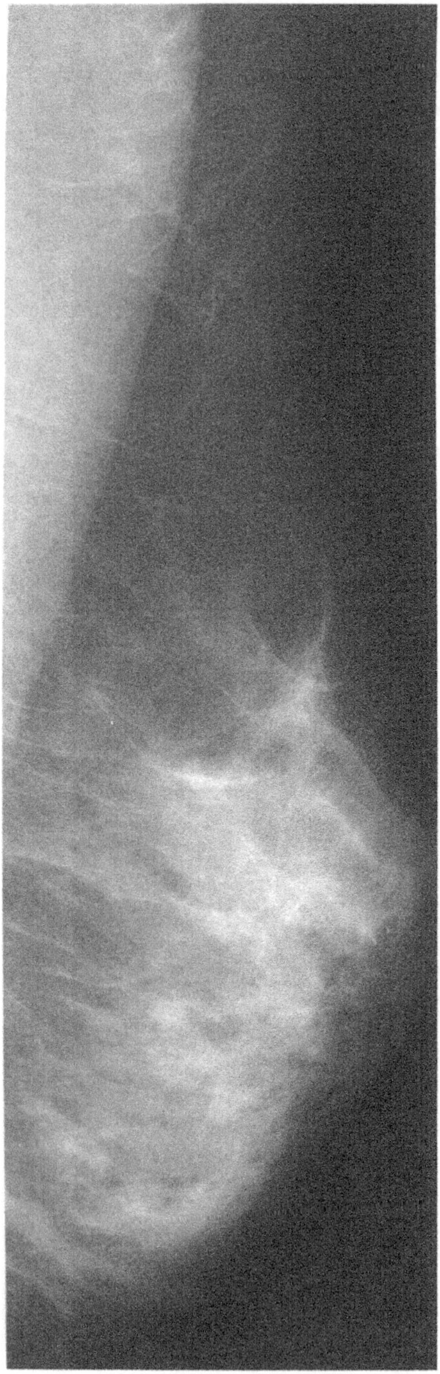

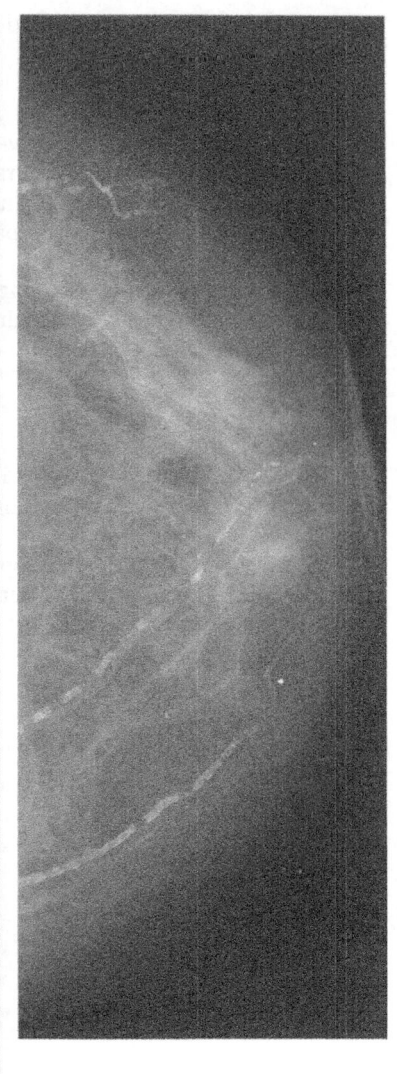

Axillary gland (lateral view).

The overall contrast is less marked in this mammogram than in Fig. 1, where the adipose tissue is particularly developed.

In the case shown here the breast is rather fibrous, with multiple images of nodular fibrosis.

The connective tissue is well developed; in the upper part of the left breast in particular there is no rupture in the architecture (*1*).

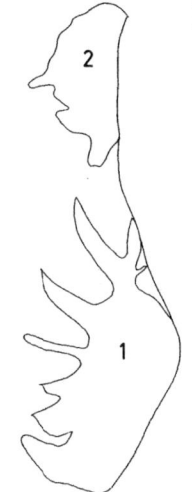

An opacity is seen in the upper part along the latissimus dorsi muscle (*2*); it shows the same radiographic characteristics as the connective supporting tissue of the breast proper. It is an accessory mammary gland in the axillary position, a real embryologic vestige. Awareness of the existence of axillary glands is extremely useful, since they exhibit the same pathologic changes as the mammary gland and undergo the same cyclic modifications as the normal breast. Hence, the interest in performing views of the axillary prolongation, which are the only ones to permit this diagnosis.

A postmenopausal breast with marked infiltration of the adipose tissue. **4** Interpretation becomes easier, since pathologic changes are more readily recognized.

Note the presence of typically vascular calcifications without mammary specificity, since they can be found in any parenchyma.

Note also the perfect tangential position of the nipple on this AP view.

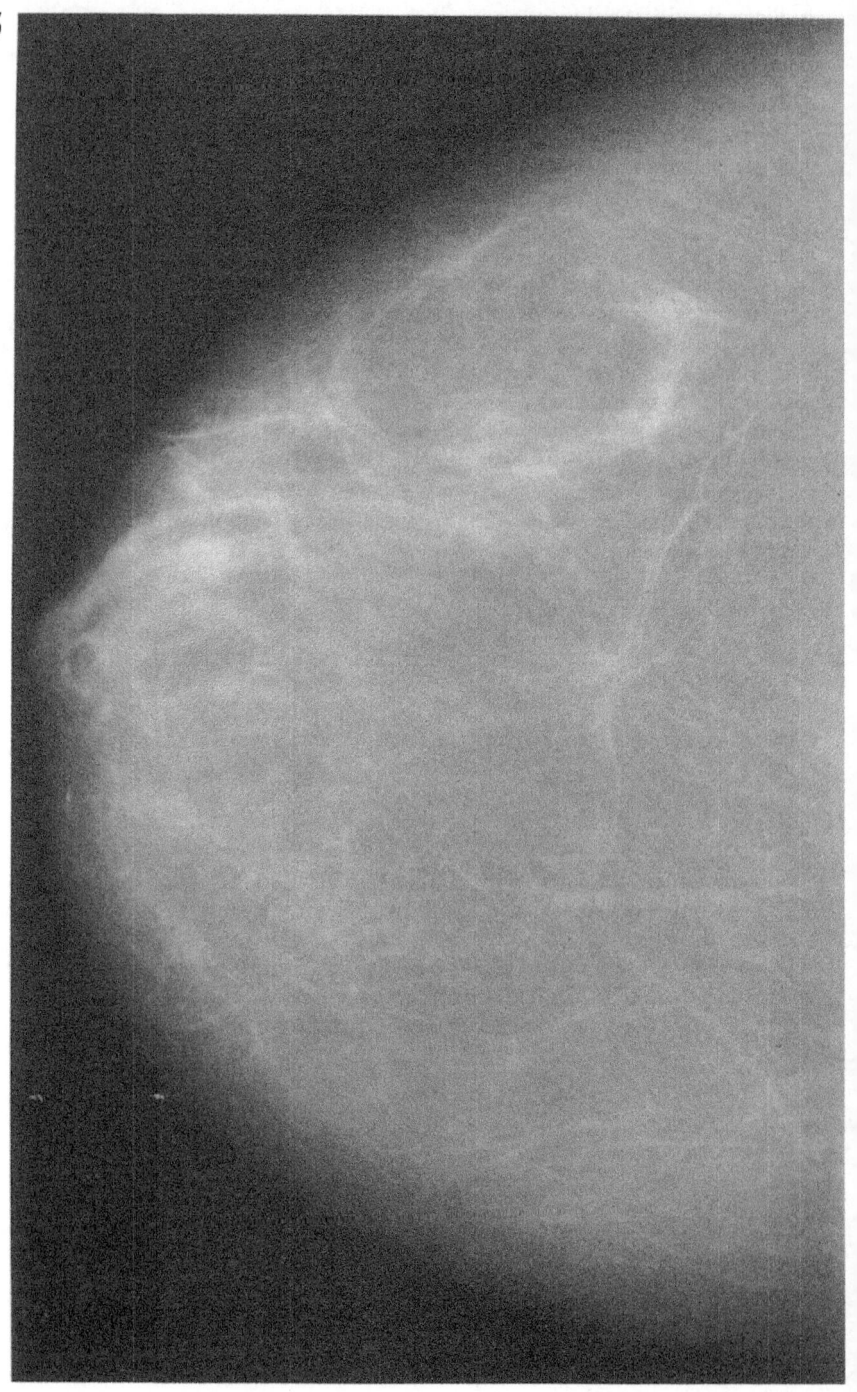

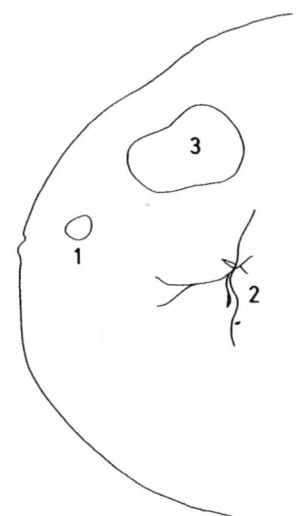

Adipose breast with postmenopausal appearance. The fibrous structures are well outlined.

Several abnormalities are visible:

1. Oval, dense, homogeneous, and well-delimited opacity in the retromamillary area in a slightly lateral situation (*1*); here and there superimposition of lucent images which correspond to ductal ectasia. The rounded opacity corresponds to a fibromatous-type lesion.

2. Posteriorly, in the deeper part of the breast, an architectural rupture seen as a linear fibrous opacity (*2*), perpendicular to the other structures.

3. In the lateral area, a hyperlucent image, visible only because it is individualized with regard to the remaining breast tissue by an opaque shell (*3*).

This is the typical image of a lipoma.

6

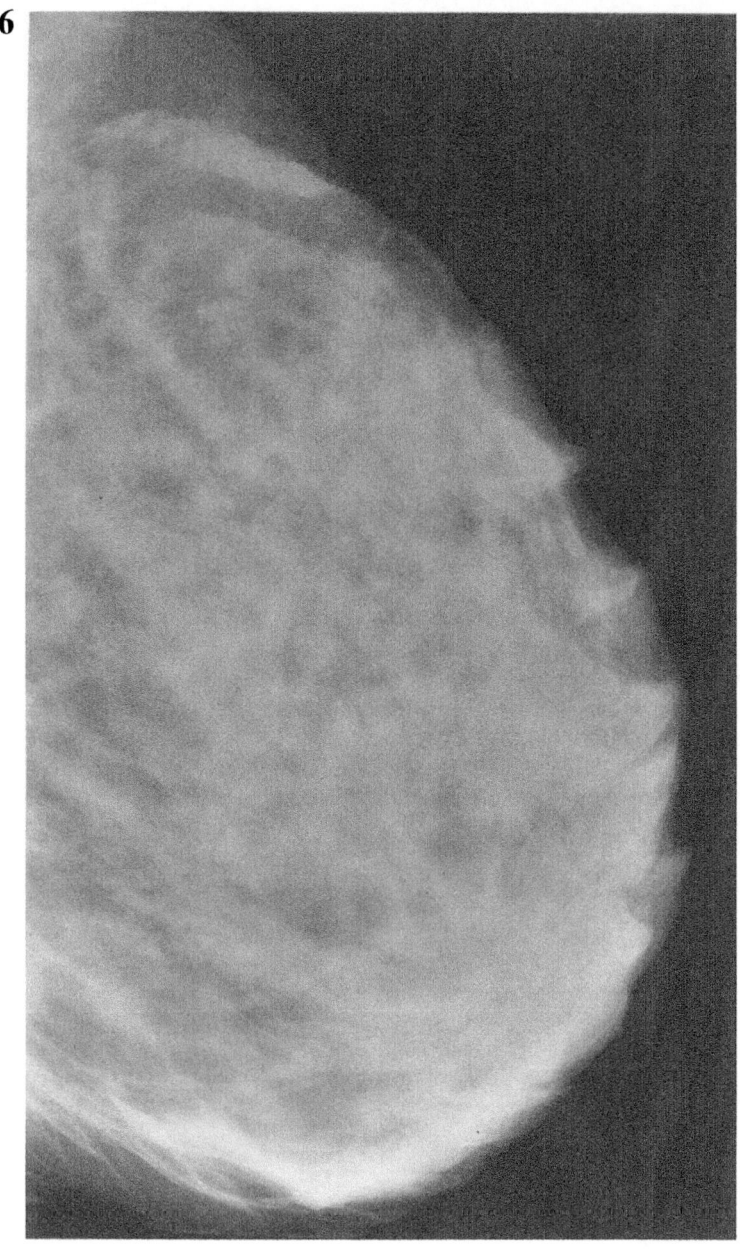

Lateral view. Normal breast with normal fibroglandular distribution. **6**

The thick opaque images on the anterior and inferior border of the breast correspond to the mammary crests. Anatomically, these crests (Duret's crests) are expansions of the fibrous tissue which cover the glandular structures and attach them to the dermis. The crests are often vascularized and show vascular swelling during the premenstrual period, sometimes even a clinically palpable nodule. In the upper region of the breast there is a plaque of encapsulated fibrosis.

A Duret's crest which is clinically palpable should always be examined with a centered radiograph. Small cancerous lesions at their onset may have a similar appearance.

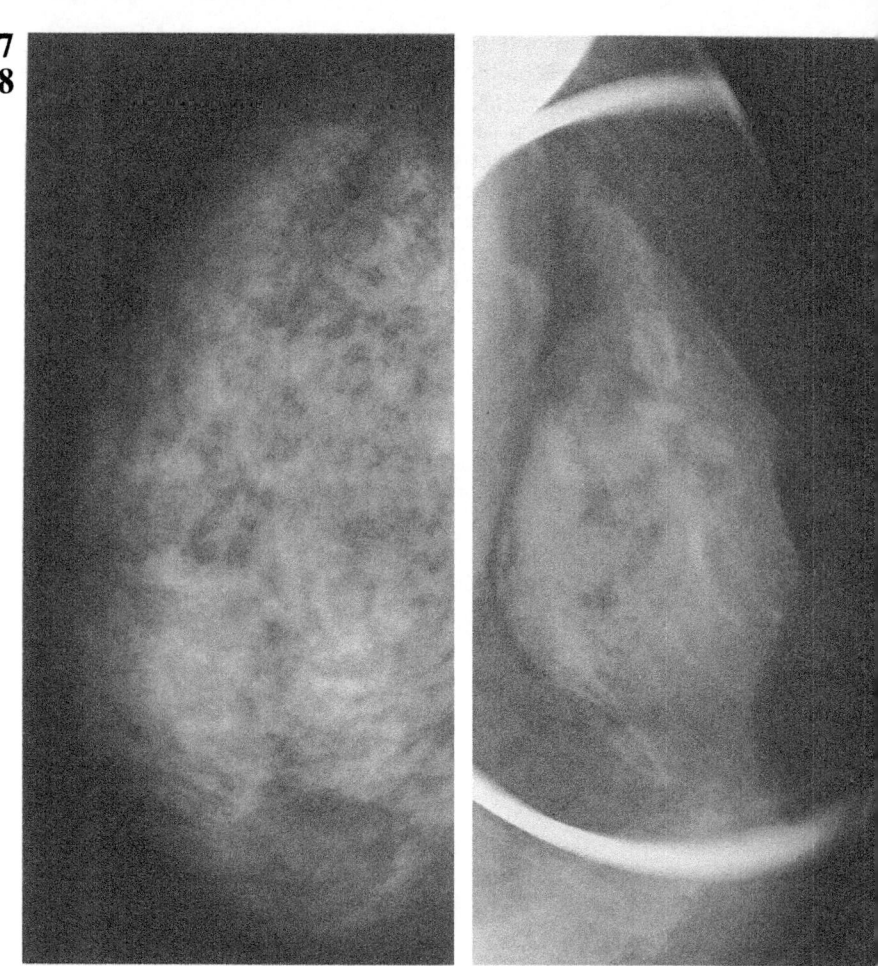

7   **8**

Lateral view. This breast is clearly different from the transparent breast shown in **7**
Fig. 1–5.

It is much more dense, with multiple nodular structures which are all regular, of the same size, and without rupture in their orientation. These nodular images correspond to elements of fibrosis, and the radiographic appearance is that of nodular fibrosis.

Early stages of degenerative lesions are not easily visualized in these structures. Therefore, any clinical abnormality should be an indication for centered radiographs.

Normal variant. Well-defined opacity with regard to adjacent structures. A radiograph centered on this palpable mass shows a fairly dense and homogeneous opacity, perfectly delineated anteriorly and posteriorly. 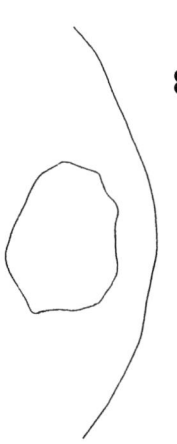 **8**

Some fibrous superimpositions on the upper and lower poles are due to the adjacent breast tissue.

Histologically, the encapsulated opacity corresponds to a plaque of fibrosis. Note that these plaques of fibrosis almost always have a rectilinear and relatively geometric appearance.

This image corresponds to localized fibrous dystrophy.
At this point it may be useful to recall the difference between dystrophy and dysplasia:

– Dystrophy is a disturbance in the vascularization and nutrition of the tissue, responsible for architectural changes.
– Dysplasia is a disturbance in the cellular growth, leading to proliferative and ill-structured tissue development.

9
10

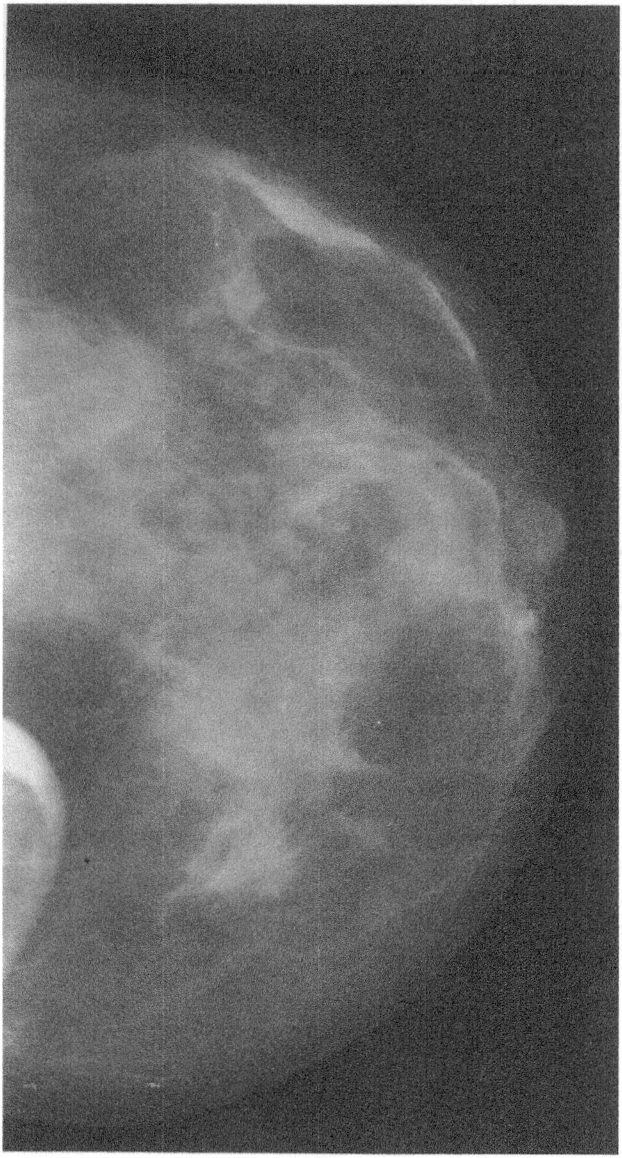

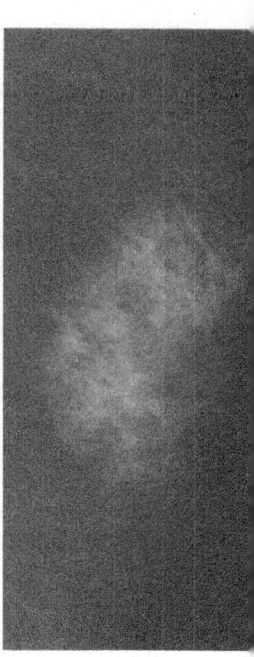

10

9   **Int.**

12

Harmonious breasts with a perfect balance of the adipose and fibroglandular **9** tissues. This radiograph shows a lateral curvilinear opacity. This image is one of the classical pitfalls associated with craniocaudal projections. It is, in fact, the auricle of the patient's ear.

Development of a dendritic opacity corresponding to a glandular structure in the **10** male, in the right retroareolar region, with fatty infiltration. This is the image of dendritic gynecomastia.

Gynecomastia has, roughly, two radiographic appearances, the dendritic pattern shown here, or a mammary bud, as shown in Fig. 2.

The radiographic image corresponds to smooth and harmonious development of the glandular buds and of the lactiferous ducts. Diffuse opacities are seen.

II. Diffuse Opacity

11

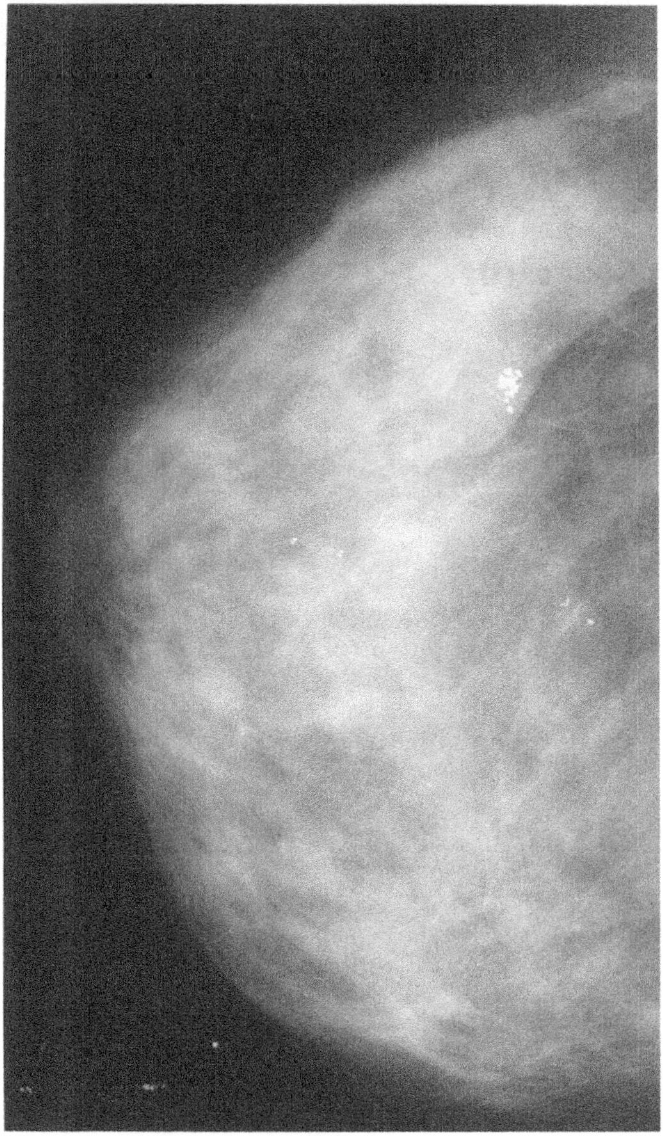

Int.

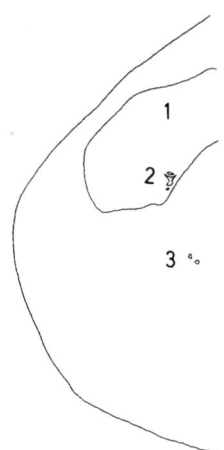

Frontal view. Relatively dense breasts with well-outlined fibrous structures, especially in the retromamillary area; the fibrous bands are harmonious, their architecture shows no disrupture.

1. A patch of fibrosis, easily recognizable due to its perfectly rectilinear delimitation, is seen in the lateral part of the right breast (*1*).
2. A group of extremely dense calcifications of equal size and homogeneous density is visible within the fibrotic patch. This image suggests an ancient fibroadenoma in the process of calcification (*2*).
3. Note some punctate or curvilinear calcifications of the same nature in the deeper central area of the breast (*3*).

Int.

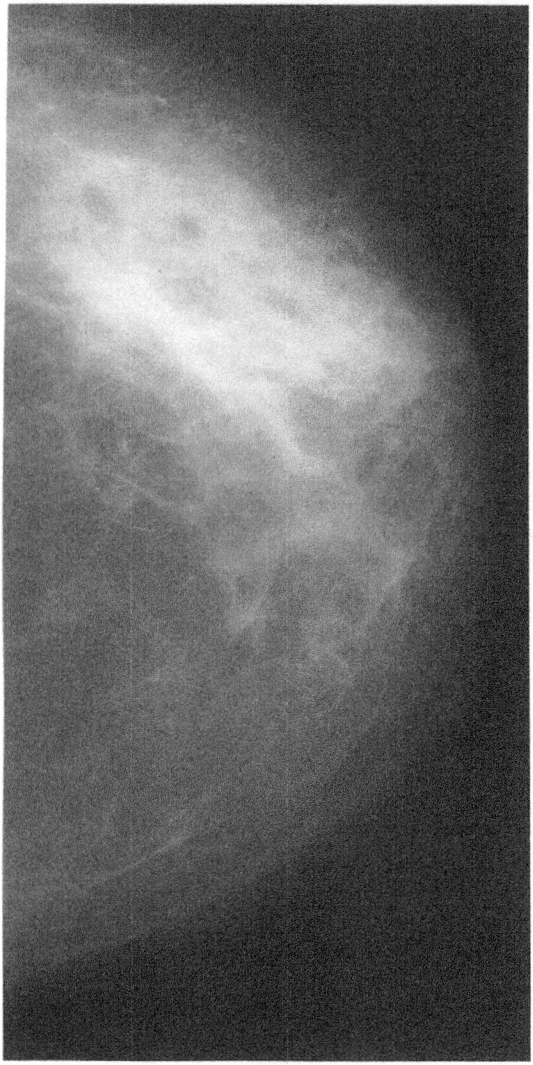

Two radiographs taken at 3 months' interval in the same patient.

On the first radiograph (**a**) note, a diffuse opacity in the lateral part of the breast. The opacity is rather homogeneous but contains some lucent areas. There is no rugged appearance and there are no irregular contours. Clinical data suggest a trivial acute inflammatory process.

18

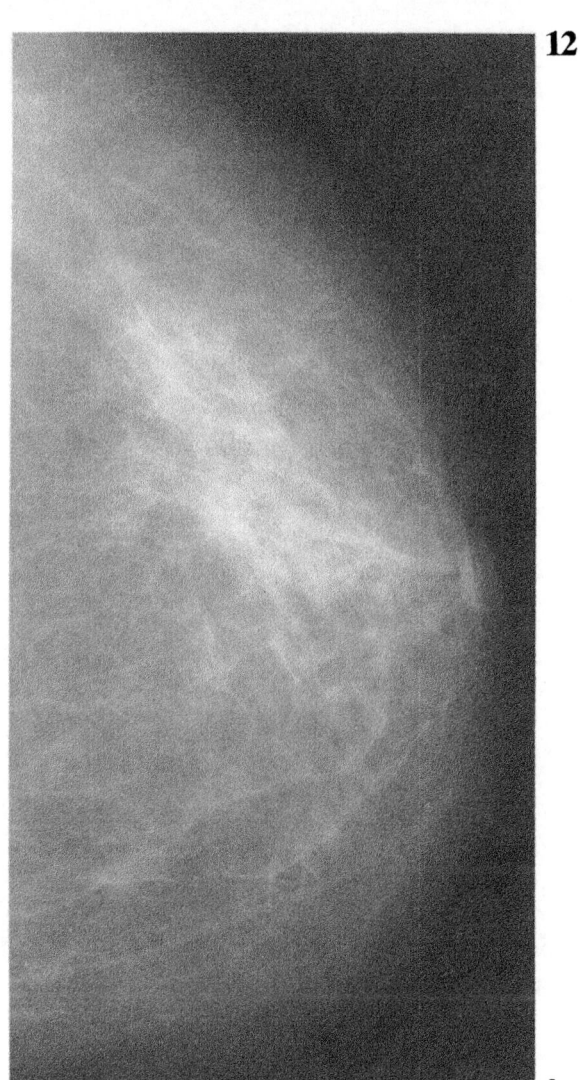

12

b

Int.

Control after antibiotic therapy (**b**) shows almost complete disappearance of the opacity, with a radiolucent breast and predominance of adipose tissue.

13
14

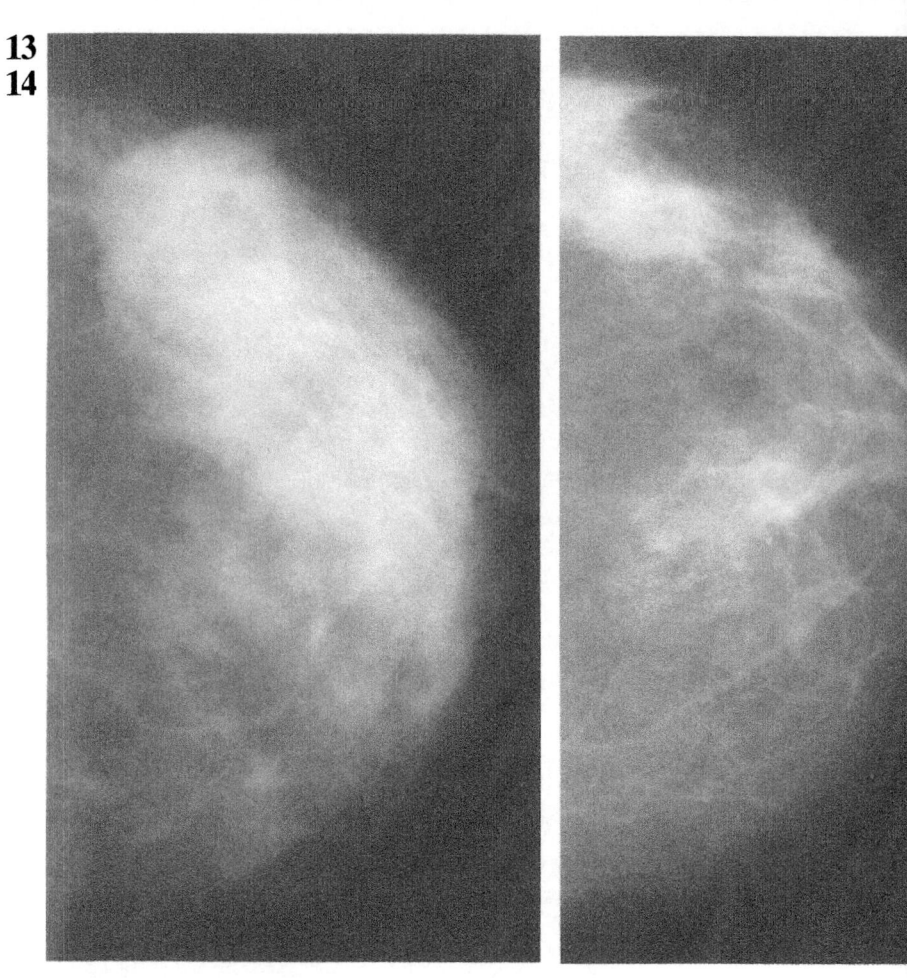

13   Int.   14   Int.

Frontal view. Note, as in Fig. 11, the presence of a large and very homogeneous patch of fibrosis in the lateral area. A closer study of the fibrotic patch shows the very irregular and rugged appearance of its lateral pole and anterior edge with divergent opacities. The patch of fibrosis, recognizable by its rectilinear margin, also contains a tumoral proliferation which consists of an infiltrating epithelioma of the lateral region.

Therefore, any patch of fibrosis should be carefully studied, and any expansion of its margins should be examined by spot films to ensure that lesions developing within a patch of fibrosis do not go undetected.

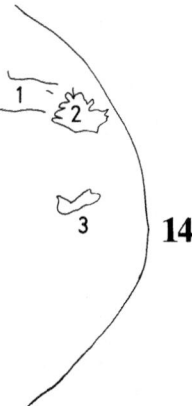

Within a lateral patch of fibrosis (*1*) note a diffuse opacity, strongly infiltrative and divergent, suggesting a proliferative process (*2*).

An opacity of the same nature can be seen, very small, and also irregular in the median retromamillary part of the breast (*3*). A histologic study performed after mammectomy revealed this to be a bifocal, lateral and medial epithelioma.

15

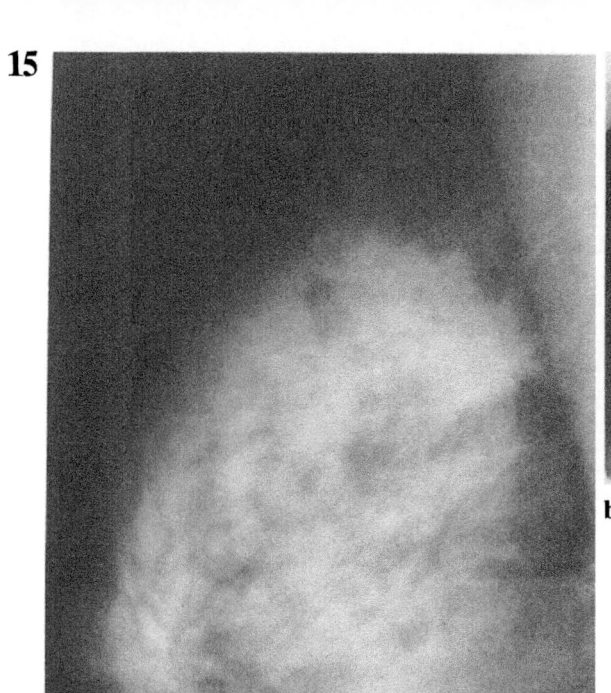

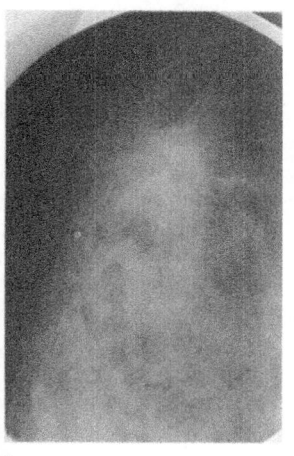

a

b

Plain radiograph (**a**) shows a fibrotic breast with numerous structures of nodular fibrosis. In the upper area of the breast, close to the muscular relief, is a ragged opacity corresponding to obvious architectural disrupture.

A view localized onto the lesion (**b**), by lowering secondary radiation, permits a better study of this image and shows clearly a radiate opacity with spicules. In front of it are small calcifications with translucent centers. They are benign.

Histology confirmed the presence of an epithelioma developing in a fibrous breast.

16

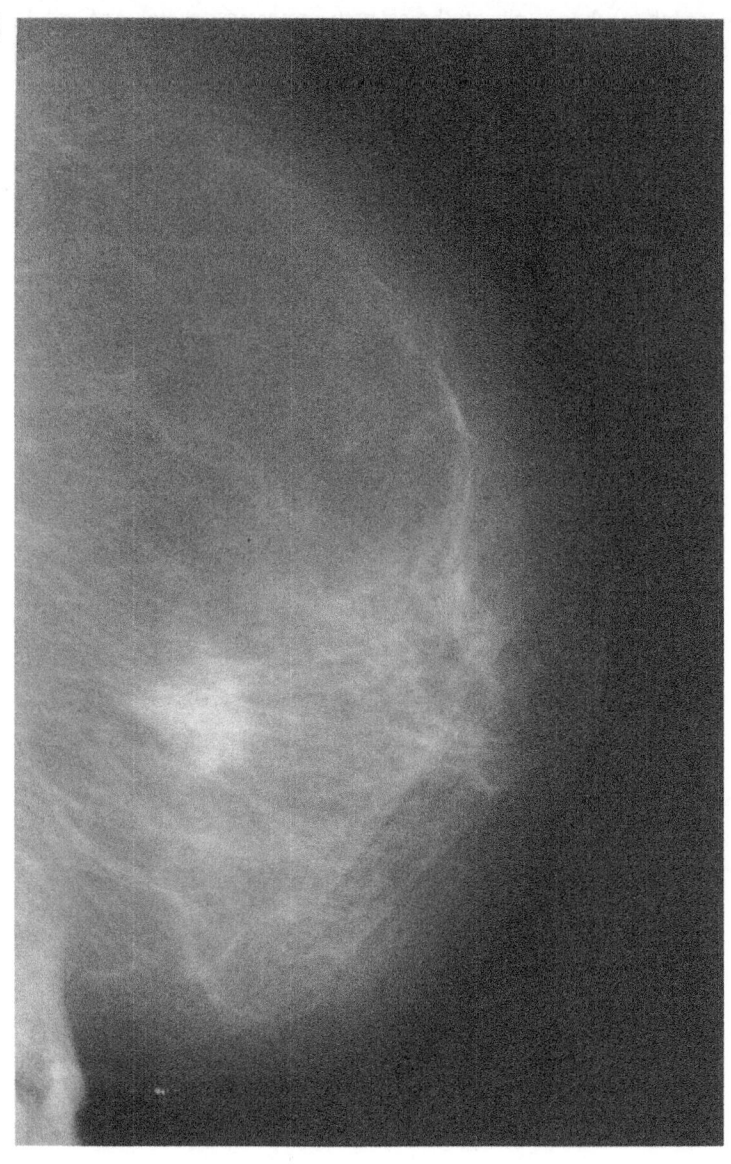

In a more clear breast, poorly delineated homogeneous opacity with ragged **16** contours is seen. The expansions of this tumor are well visible. The radiological appearance corresponds to invasion of the adjacent tissue by neoplastic cells. In this case, too, the histologic findings confirmed a strongly infiltrating diffuse lactiferous epithelioma, without stromal reaction. In the lower retroareolar area are multiple parallel linear opacities, corresponding to cutaneous folds.

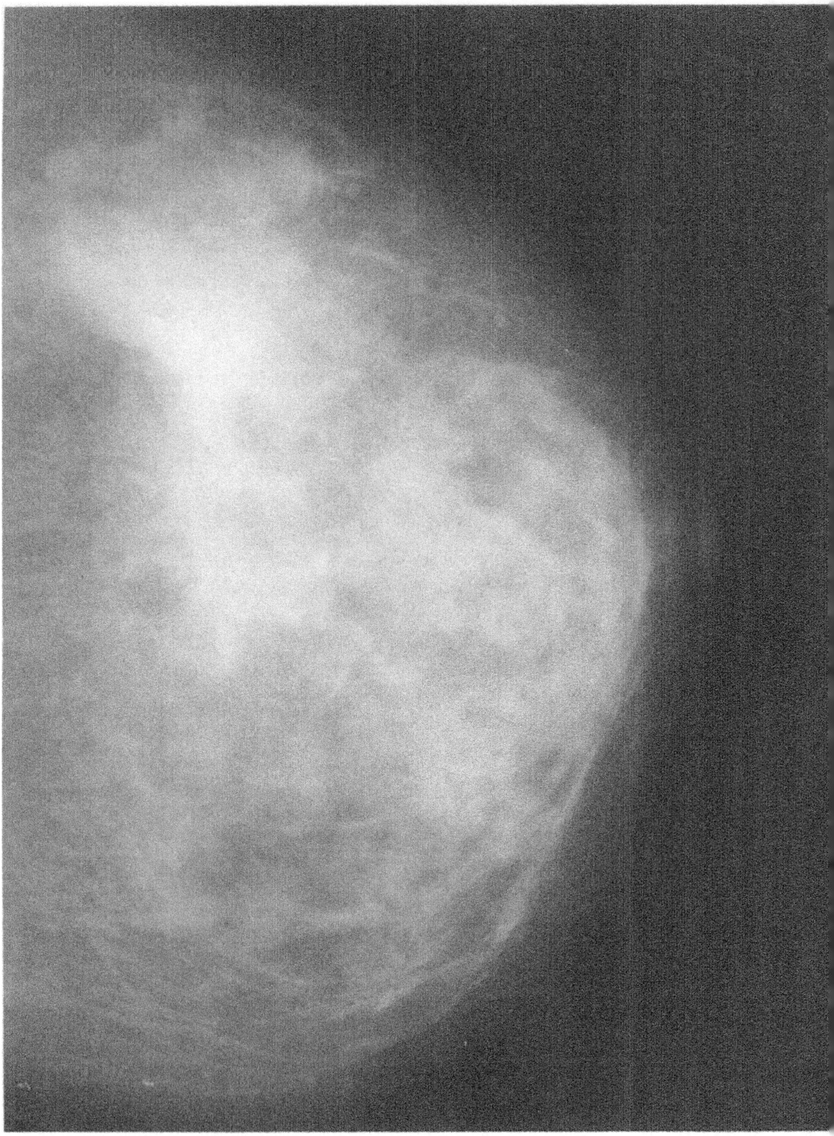

a   **Int.**

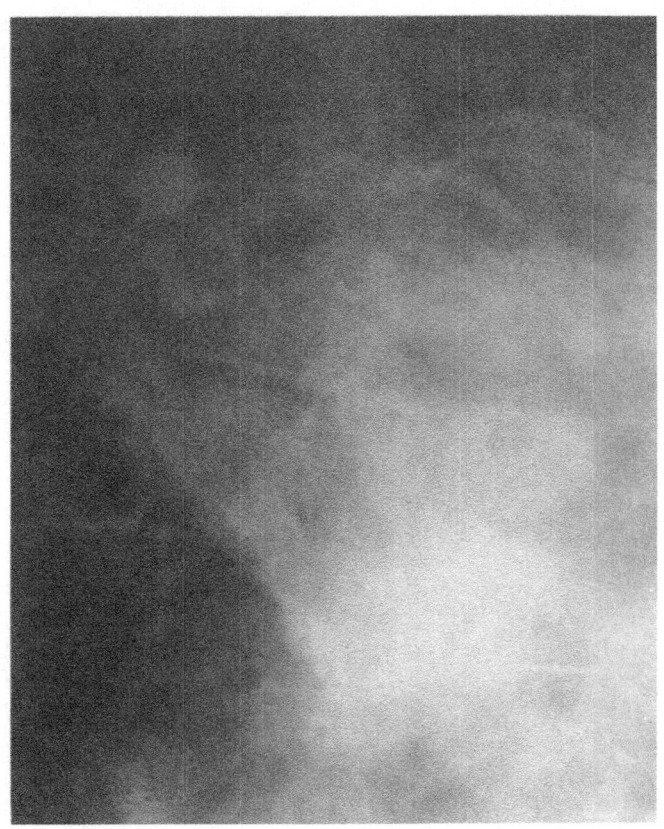

b

A poorly defined opacity with obvious disrupture in the structural organization of the tissue, disturbing the overall harmony of the breast (**a**).

The magnified spot film (**b**) shows perfectly the important expansive and infiltrating opacity which corresponds to an undifferentiated invasive lactiferous epithelioma (*1*). Also note on the spot film a rounded regular opacity, corresponding to a small cutaneous tumor (*2*).

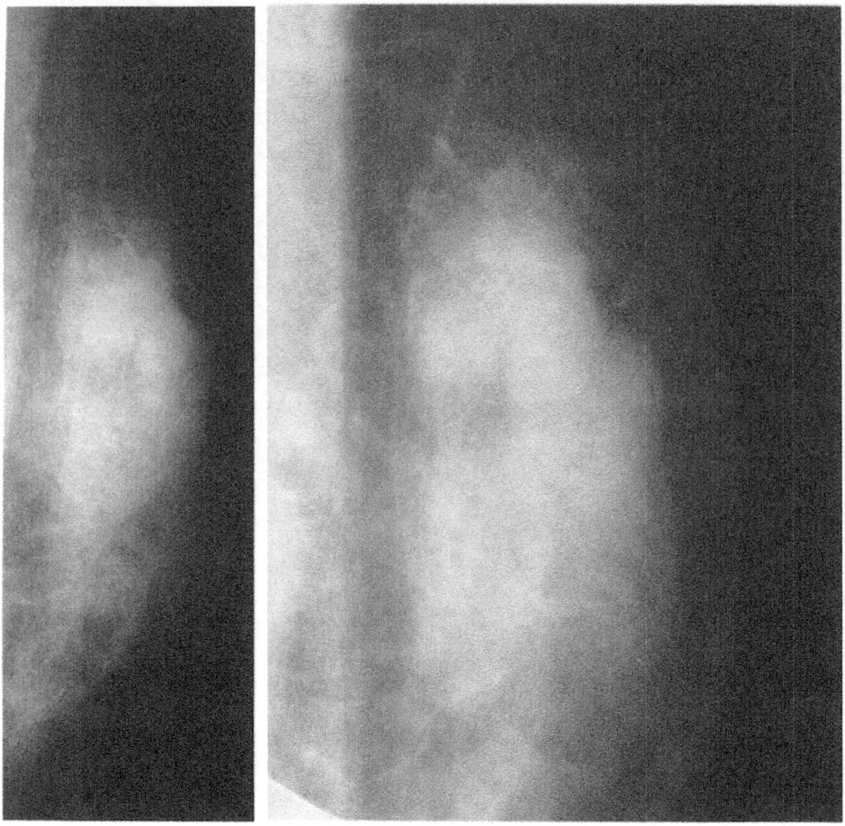

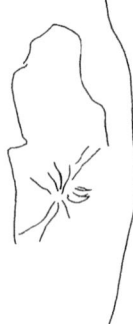

a   b

A plain radiography (**a**) shows a rather dense breast. In the upper part are several homogeneous opacities, and an area of architectural disrupture; the latter is well visualized in the magnified spot film (**b**). The opacities join to form an extended patch in the upper part of the supra-areolar region. Within this patch, the convergence image corresponds to marked stromal reaction.

Cytology confirmed a diffuse epithelioma.

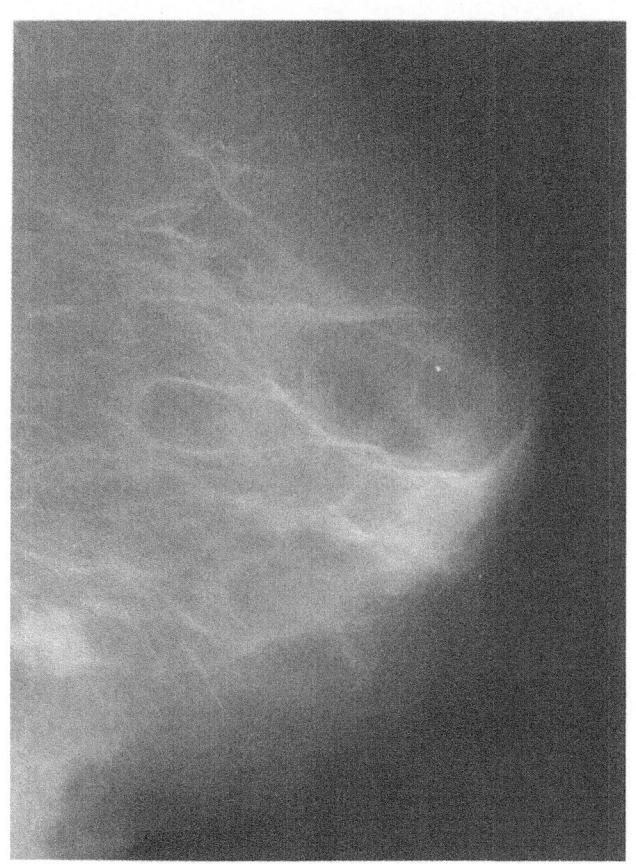

Opacity in the deep lower region in a rather clear breast. The opacity is homogeneous but its contours are irregular and poorly defined. Here and there, the opacity is prolonged by marked outgrowths.

Palpation of the lesion was difficult, because of the clinical context. The suspicious radiographic appearance led to performance of a partial mastectomy; cytology confirmed a lactiferous epithelioma without any stromal reaction.

20

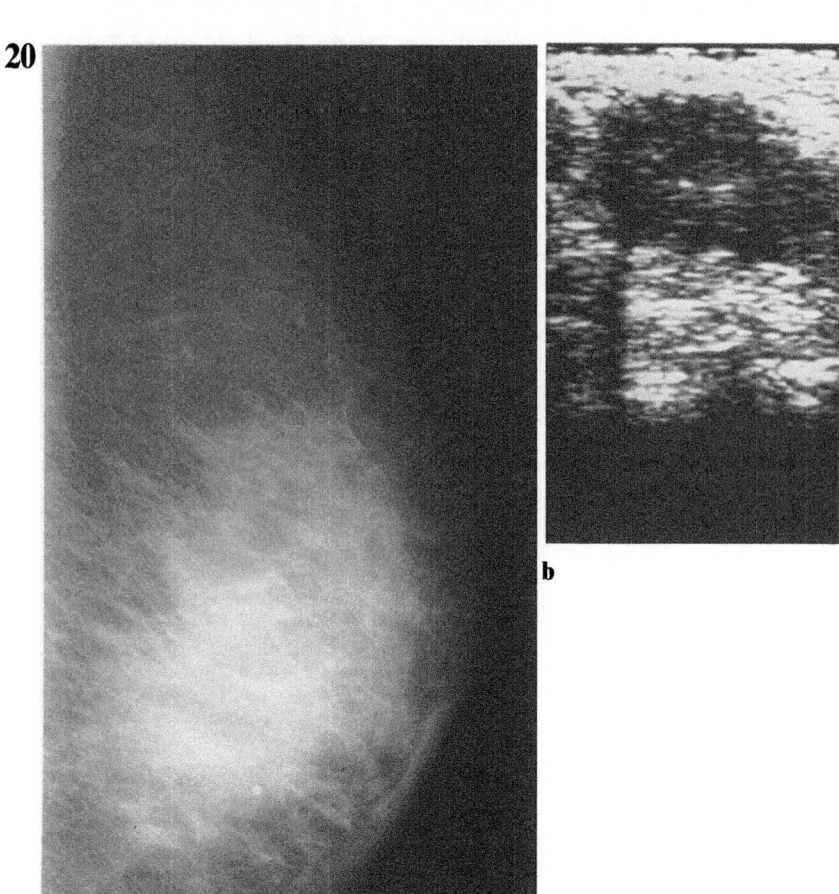

a

b

The lateral view (**a**) shows a quite extended and diffuse opacity with numerous **20** irregular expansions. Thickening of the skin in the subareolar area is a further element leading to the diagnosis of diffuse cancer. This diagnosis was confirmed by ultrasonography (**b**), which shows an irregular, lacunar image with lateral attenuation images.

Disruptures in the structural organization of the tissue are seen.

III. Architectural Rupture or Starshaped Opacities

21

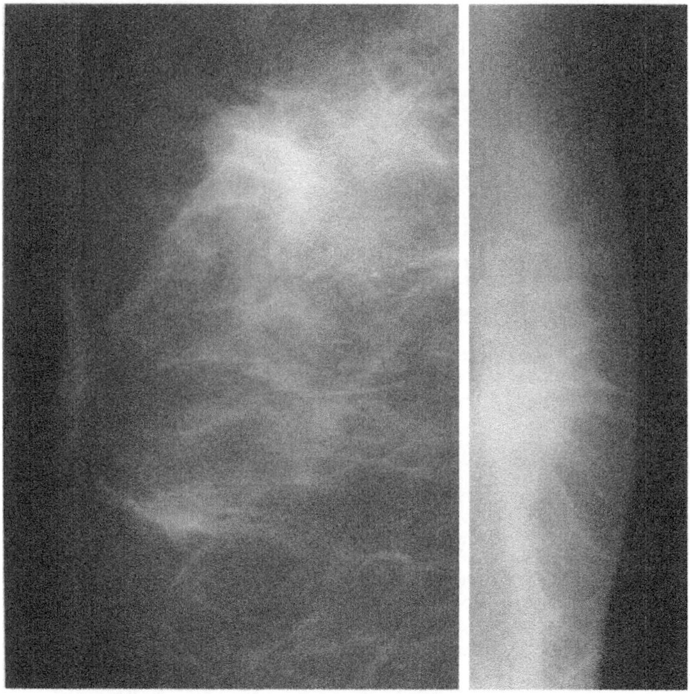

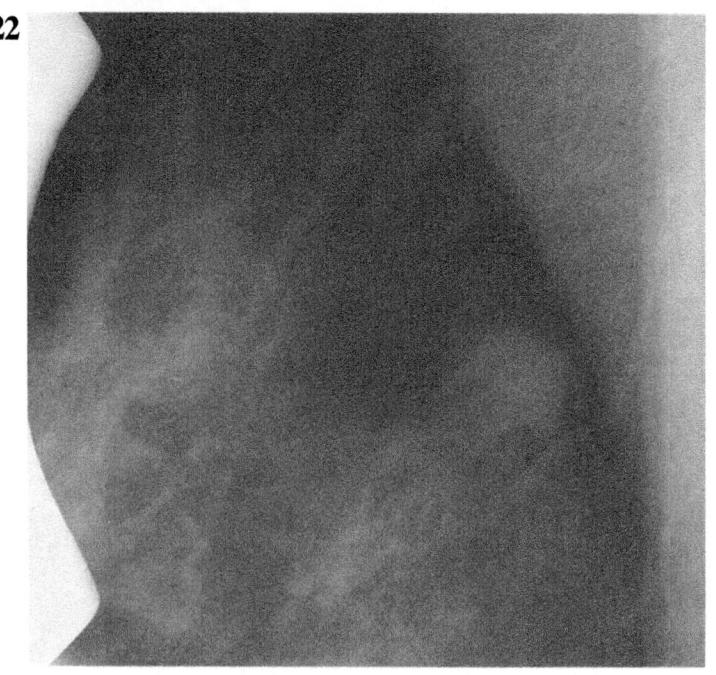

a
b

22

In a deformed breast with retraction of the nipple, an opacity is seen in the upper **21** region, corresponding to a patch of fibrosis. From this patch arise divergent linear opacities infiltrating the adjacent mammary tissues. Below the opacity there is a large number of small calcifications of markedly polymorphous and heterogeneous density. Their distribution is quite irregular, or even anarchic (**a**).

The view covering the axillary part of the breast (**b**) permits a good evaluation of the radiate linear opacities, which appear to be thicker near the tumoral opacity than at the periphery. Indeed, the farther from the tumor, the purer the fibrosis (stromal reaction). Close to the tumor the image corresponds to the junction of the cancerous spicules (groups of invading cancer cells) and the reactional fibrosis.

These radiographs correspond to an epithelioma which is mainly intracanalar and has developed on a patch of fibrosis.

Magnified spot film of a deep-lying opacity, close to the muscular plane. The **22** opacity is slightly dense and has markedly irregular contours. This is the radiographic appearance of a poorly cellular but strongly infiltrating cancer (lobular epithelioma).

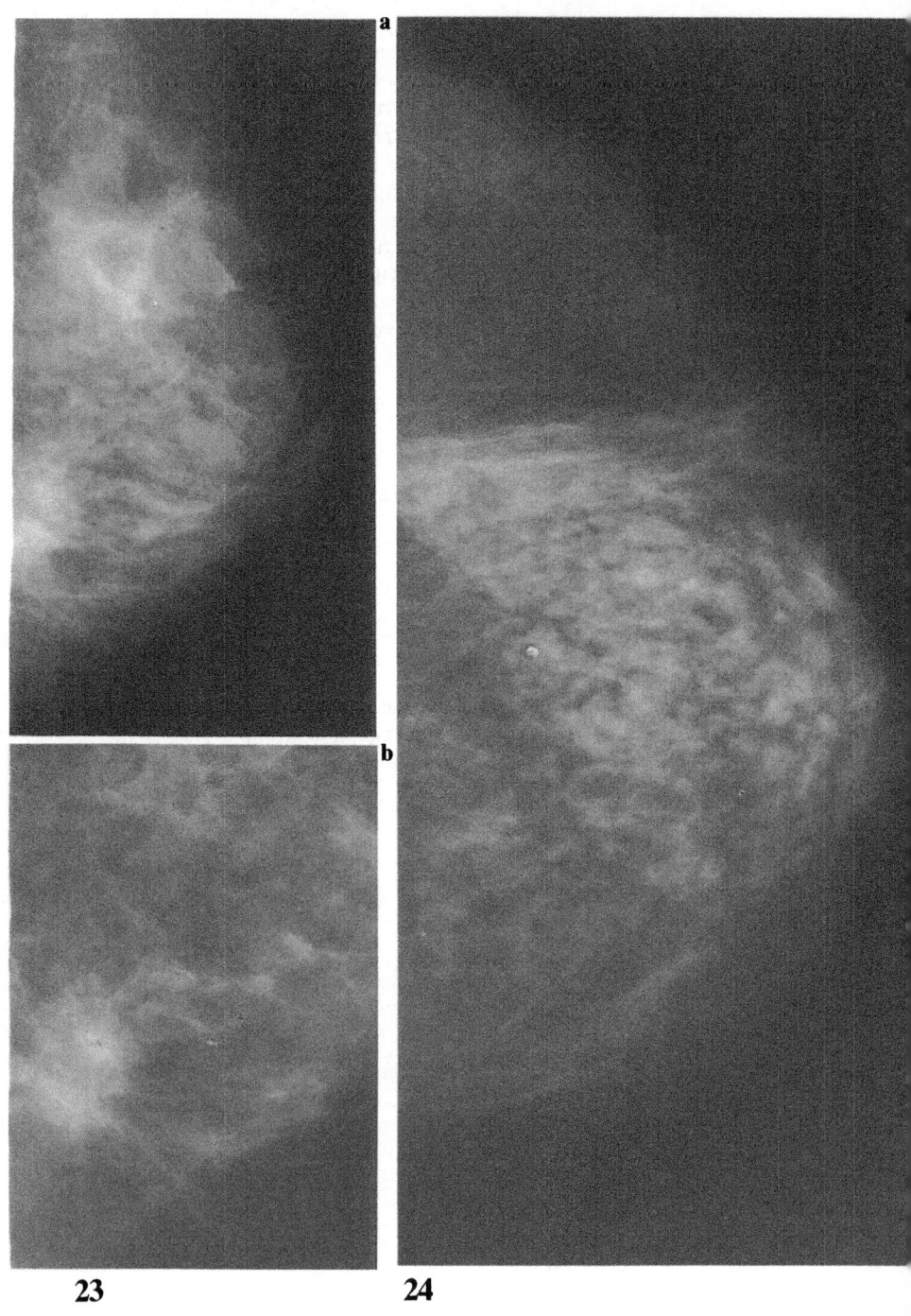

23

24

Irregular opacity in the right lower quadrant (**a**). The spot film (**b**) shows the **23** opacity to have irregular expansions, to a much greater extent than would have been suspected from the plain radiographs. In fact, the expansions reach the subcutaneous layer. In this case, too, the image of architectural rupture corresponds to that of an epithelioma with marked stromal reaction.

The entire lateral part of the left breast appears void compared with the rest of **24** the breast, which contains nodular fibrosis elements. The transparent structure, visible only because it is delineated by the surrounding densification, corresponds to a lipoma.

Note also, in the deeper retroareolar area, the presence of a calcification with a clear center (cytosteatonecrosis).

25

Int.

Int.

Int.

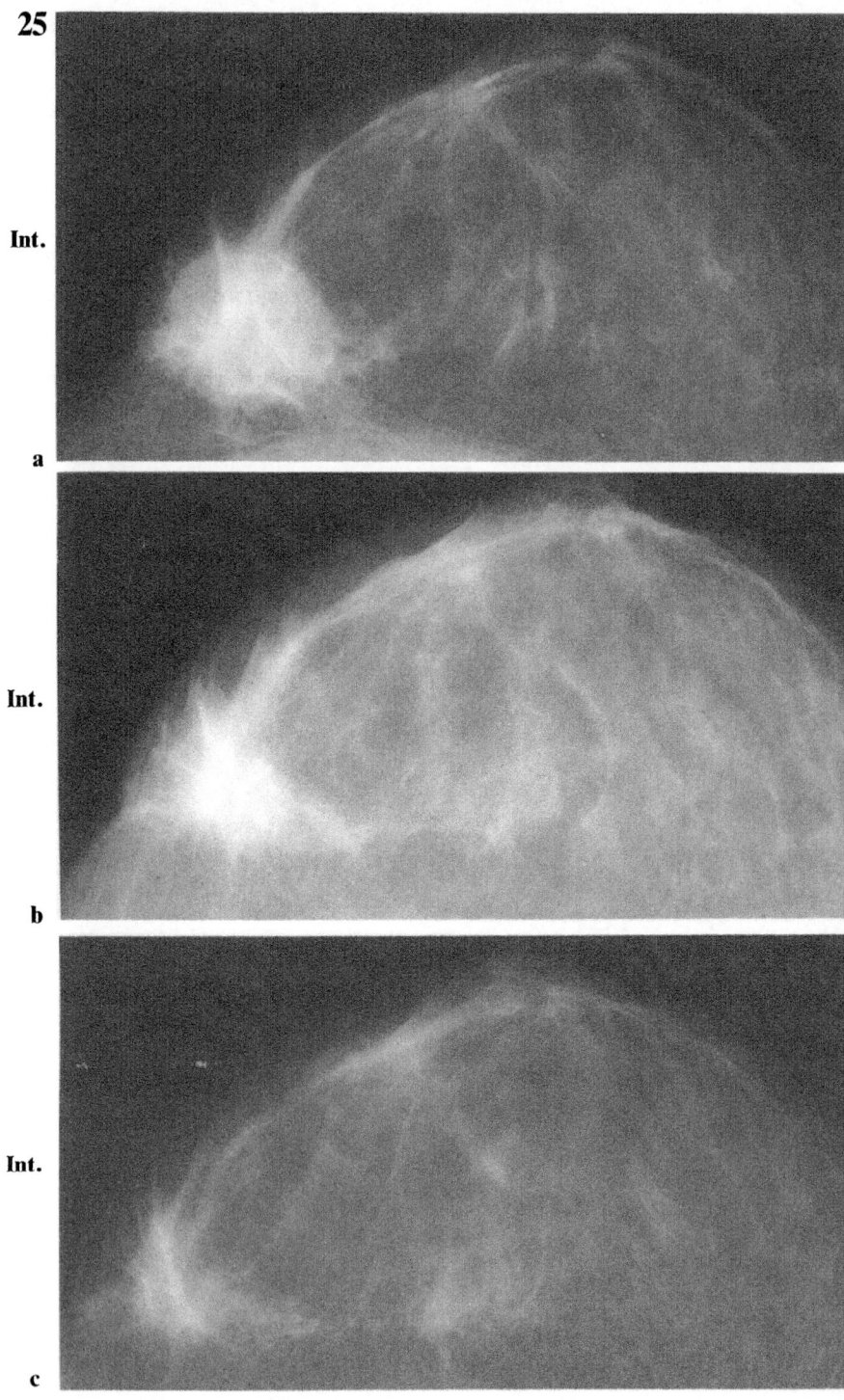

a

b

c

Three successive radiographs performed in a patient who had undergone surgery a few days before the first was taken for a benign fibroadenomatous lesion.

The opacity is dense, homogeneous, and well delineated, but there are some branching divergent linear opacities, as well as discrete retraction. The diagnosis was hematoma, but a control was advised after a short interval because of a stellate image in the lateral region.

Two months later, the opacity has almost entirely disappeared. The marked structural disruption persists, but there is no clinically palpable nodule.

Three months later, the stellate opacity has regressed, and the further development confirms the absence of tumoral lesion.

This case illustrates well the difficulty of a differential diagnosis between cancer and scarring. In this particular case the follow-up has confirmed the benignity. The stellate image is merely that of scarring following tumorectomy.

One can legitimately question on what grounds follow-up rather than exeresis was advised:

1. At the beginning the regressive hematoma masked the suspect image.
2. Once the hematoma had disappeared, the image had no clinical correlation. One can reasonably estimate that, if there had been a cancer, then considering the size of the suspect image there would also have been clinical signs.
3. Therefore, a last control after a short interval was recommended. It showed regular and progressive regression of the abnormal appearances.

26

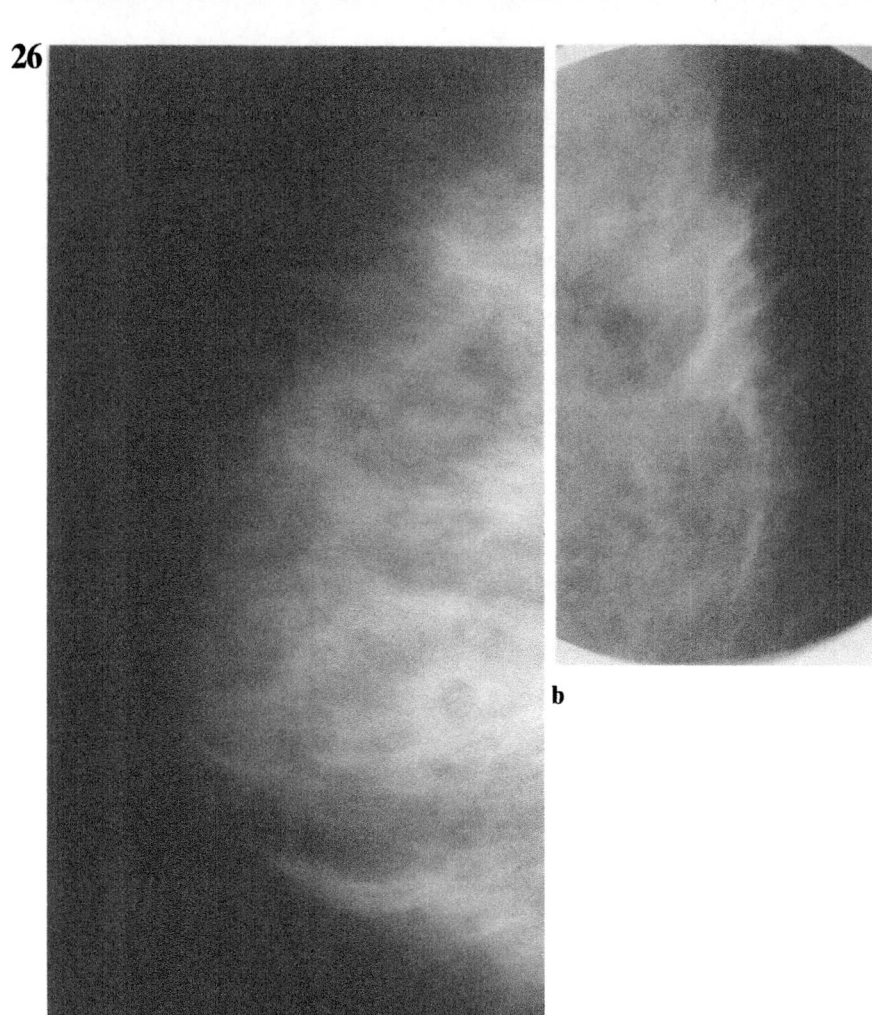

a

b

Very opaque breasts with a denser, rounded opacity in the upper area (**a**). The
appearance of this breast is characterized mainly by total rupture in its harmony.

The spot film (**b**) shows the tumoral opacity, its marked ramous prolongations, and, finally, retraction.

The histological investigation showed a highly infiltrative diffuse epithelioma.

27

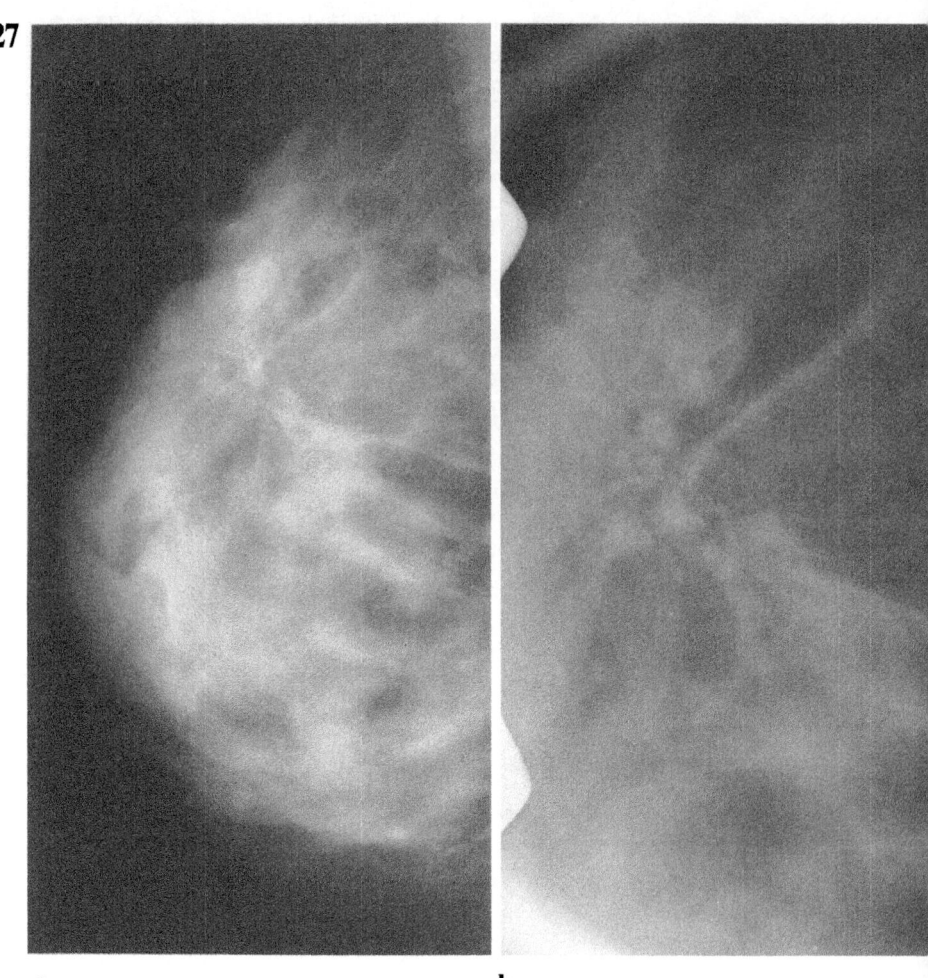

a   b

The entire upper part of the breast is the site of retraction remodeling without individualized tumoral opacity (**a**). The enlarged spot film (**b**) confirms the absence of tumoral opacity but clearly demonstrates the presence of divergent fibrous opacities. This image points up the problem of differential diagnosis with cancer lesions; nothing on this radiograph permits ruling out the presence of a carcinoma, of which the only mammographic sign would be stroma reaction.

However, the absence of a palpable nodule, although there are marked alterations, and also the absence of any direct sign of malignity suggest the diagnosis of sclerosing adenosis. Radiologically, nothing in fact allows a differentiation between sclerosing adenosis and carcinoma. Surgical excision is required in any case.

In the present case, cytology confirmed the diagnosis of benign sclerosing adenosis.

28

Int.

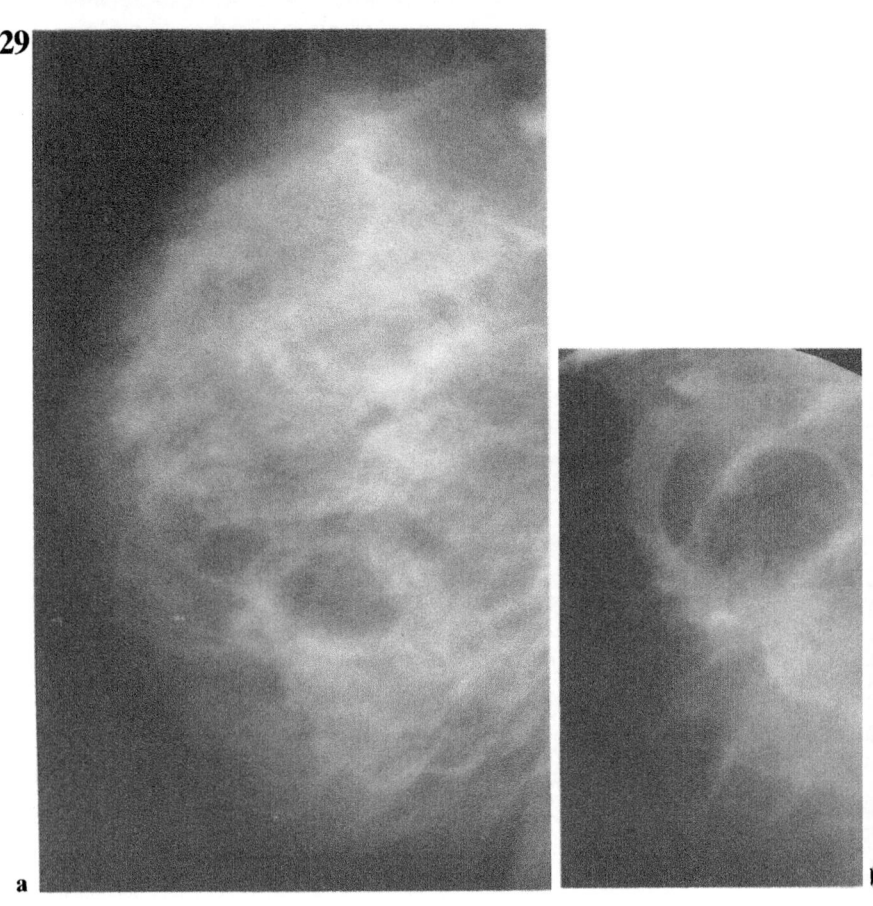

29

a

Complete disruption in the structural organization of the tissue in a breast which **28** has undergone surgical reduction. The clear retroareolar area is a result of the displacement of the areola-nipple area.

Two rather rounded and well-delimited areas are seen in the lower part of the **29** breast. The connective tissue between these two areas is more dense. The spot film demonstrates the presence of a retractile, expansive lesion.

The image is consistent with that of a very small carcinoma, less than 4 mm in diameter.

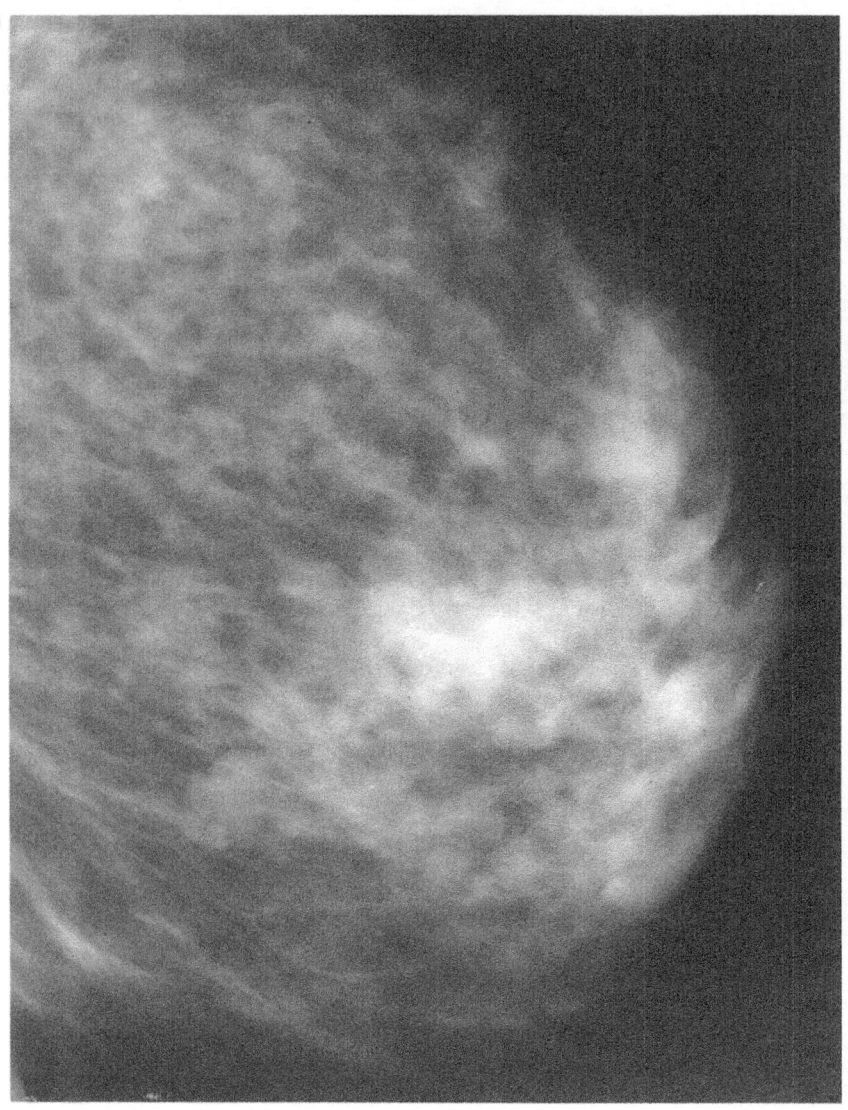

a

Right and left lateral views. In a 50-year-old woman, a rather homogeneous breast with numerous bilateral opacities, some of which are rounded, regular, and well outlined.

The overall findings correspond to fibrocystic dysplasia with elements of nodular fibrosis, small adenomas, and small cysts. On the right (**a**) is a more markedly dystrophic retromammillary patch, with numerous calcifications which are alarmingly polymorphous and very irregularly distributed. On the left (**b**) is a stellate image with a markedly infiltrating architectural rupture in the upper part.

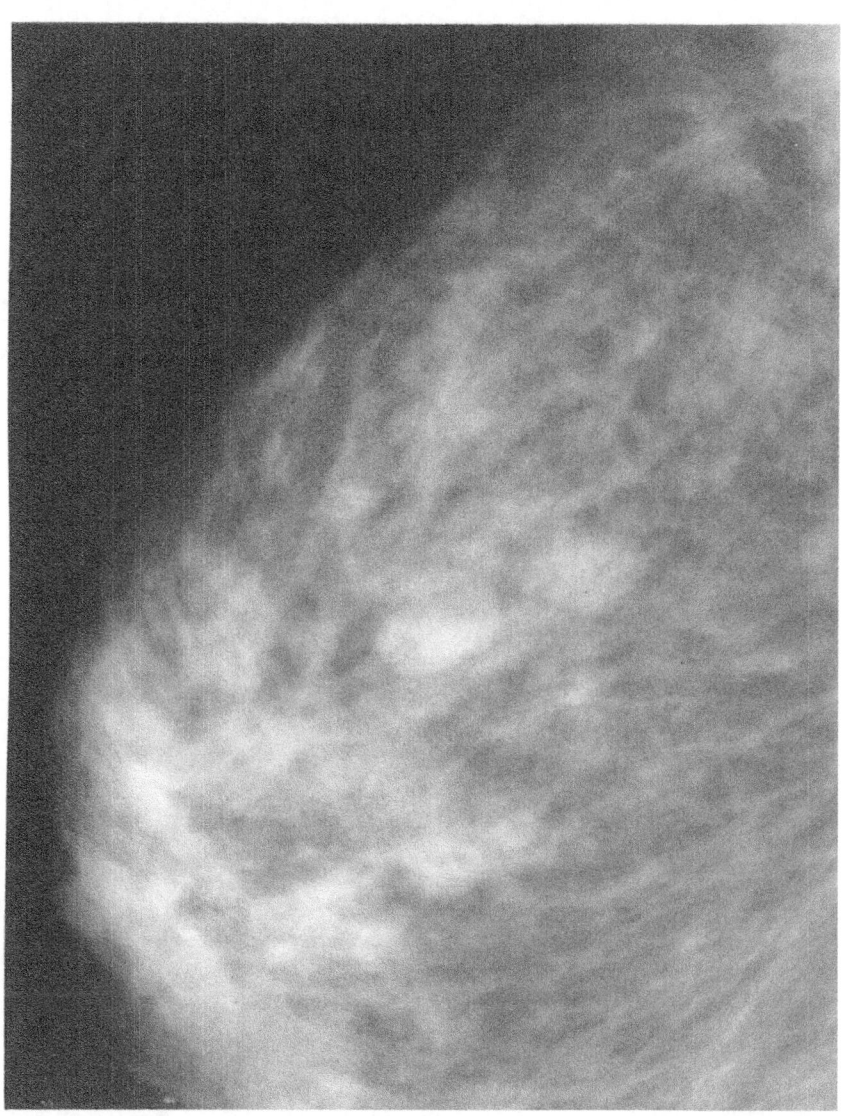

b

Because of the diffusion of the lesions and the very likely presence of a carcinoma in the left upper part, as well as the presence of suspect calcifications on the right side, a partial bilateral mammectomy was performed. This showed:
- on the right, an infiltrating epithelioma, mainly intracanalar, with additional lesions of lobular epithelioma in situ
- on the left, an infiltrating lactiferous epithelioma with a lobular epithelioma in situ

This case is a good illustration of the ambiguity of breast cancer imaging, since the same carcinomatous lesion can result in radically different images.

31

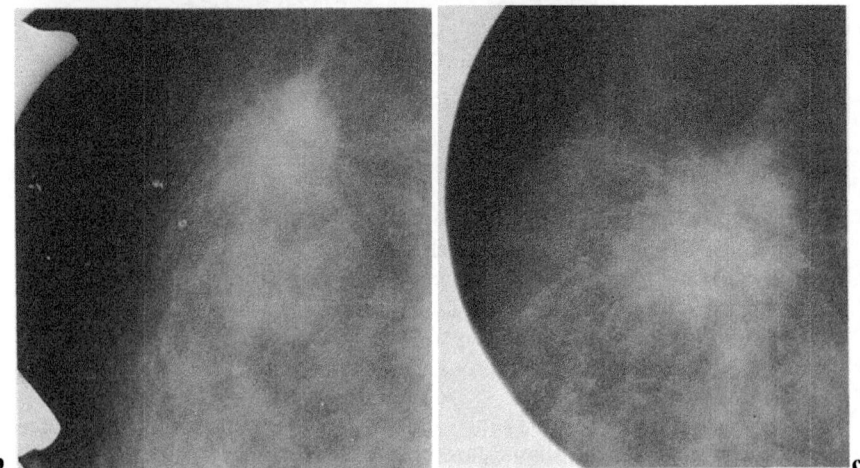

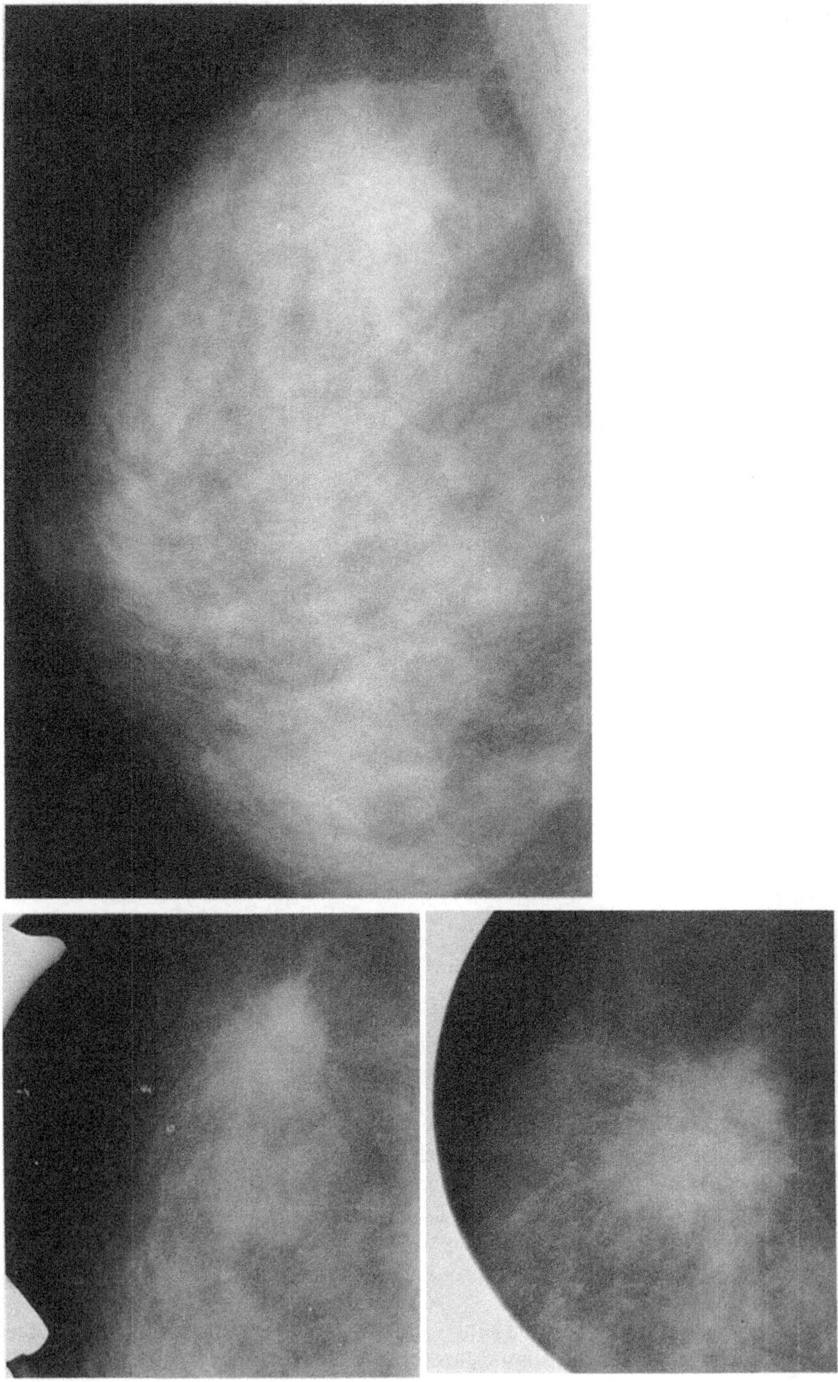

Plain radiograph (**a**) shows a fibrotic breast. A triangular patch of unimportant
fibrosis is seen in the lower part. The upper part has a heterogeneous, spiky
appearance. No conclusion can be drawn from this radiograph.

The spot view (**b**), unenlarged, shows a strongly heterogeneous opacity, with
multiple fibrous expansions and a benign calcification. The enlarged spot film (**c**)
provides a better visualization of the opacity and permits a more detailed study
of its contours. The opacity corresponds, in fact, to a small epitheliomatous
lesion with marked stromal reaction and malignant calcifications.

This case points up the value of performing spot films, with or without
magnification; due to different compression, slightly different incidence, and
especially absence of diffuse radiation, spot films allow a more precise study of
dense opacities.

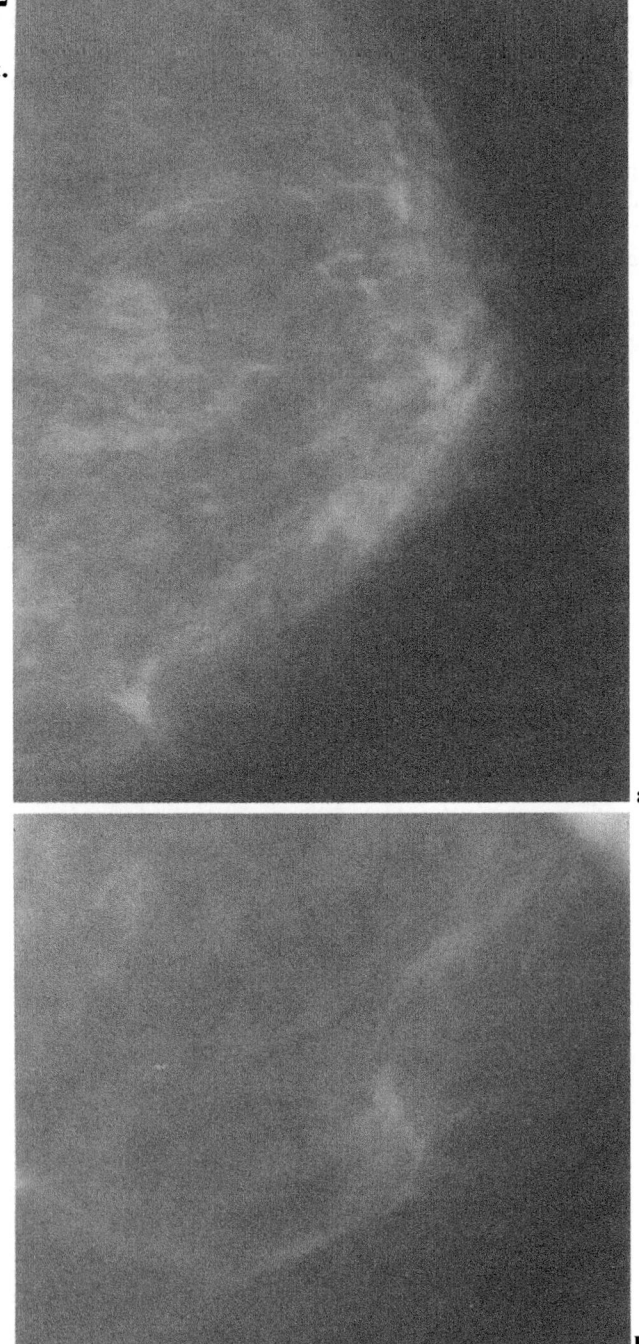

a

b

Radiograph shows obvious rupture in the structural organization of the lateral **32** part of the right breast. There is a linear opacity which is perpendicular to the remainder of the fibrous bands (**a**).

As usual, the enlarged spot film (**b**) permits a closer study of the opacity and gives evidence of extremely thin expansions. The architectural rupture is well demonstrated. Cytology confirmed an epithelioma of the lobular type.

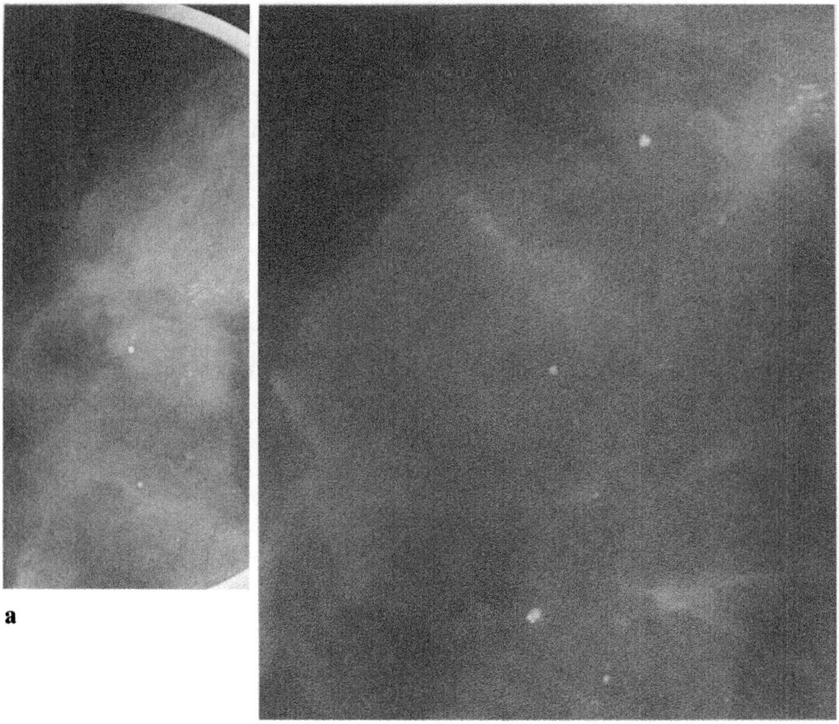

a

b

33 Spot film and enlarged spot film.

The unenlarged spot film (**a**) shows a retractile, stellate structure and behind this a group of calcifications of heterogeneous size, orientation, shape, and density.

In the upper part of the spot film other, more regular and less numerous calcifications alternate with small clusters of microcalcifications. The magnified spot film (**b**) provides a better image of the calcifications.

Cytology demonstrated the association of an infiltrating lobular type carcinoma with multiple lobular cancer lesions in situ.

34 Markedly fibrotic breasts with a clearly visible benign calcification. In the upper area, complete architectural rupture with retraction and vascular dilatation.

On a spot film with enlargement (**b**) this opacity is well delineated from the surrounding fibrous tissues. It shows an irregular and poorly delimited opacity with numerous digitations. The appearance is typical of infiltrating epithelioma. Rounded opacities are also seen.

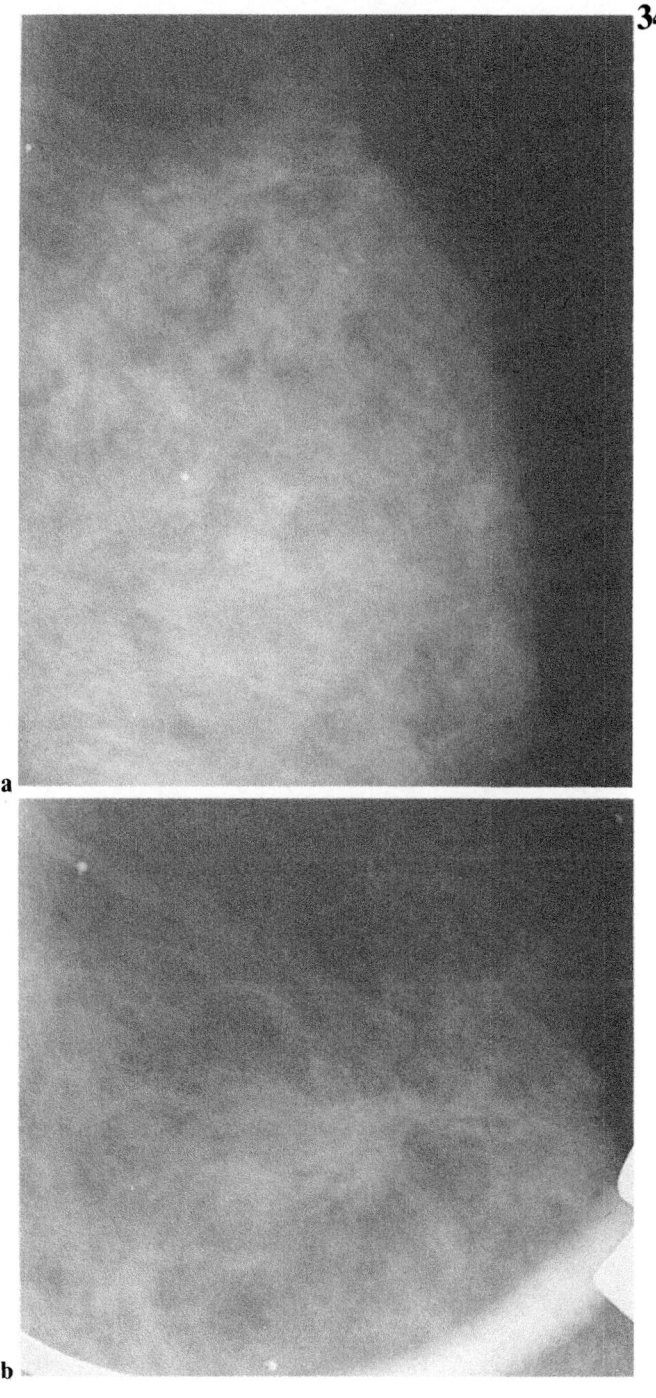

a

b

IV. Oval Opacities

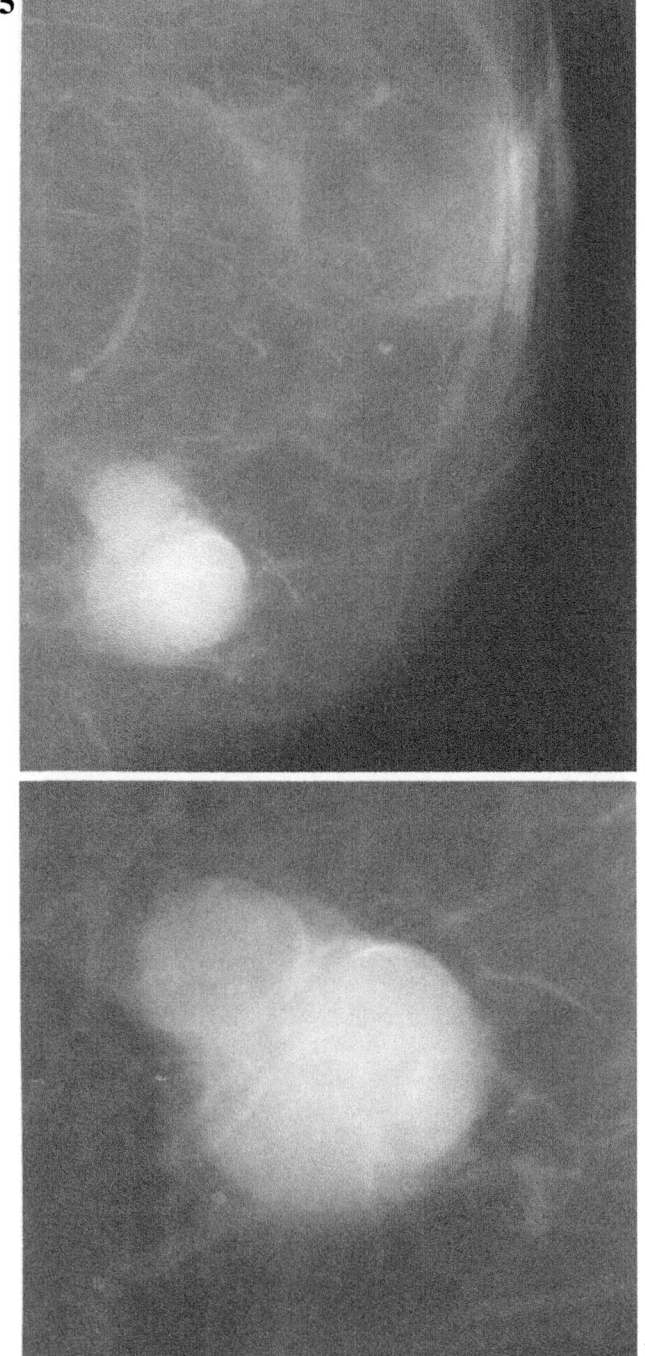

35

a

b

In this postmenopausal patient, the nodule which had led to clinical investiga- **35** tions appears on the radiographs (**a, b**) as a dense and homogeneous opacity, rather well outlined, at least as concerns its anterior contour. Posteriorly, there is a smaller opacity with a somewhat irregular contour.

This case also illustrates the ambiguity of breast radiology: a relatively regular image can correspond to colloid carcinoma as well as to a cystic structure. In the case presented, the irregularities in the posterior contour and the unsharpness of the medial part of the contour, as well as the increased caliber of a nearby vessel, suggest carcinoma. Note also the presence of a curvilinear calcification which corresponds to a benign calcification of the wall.

Cytology confirmed colloid carcinoma.

36

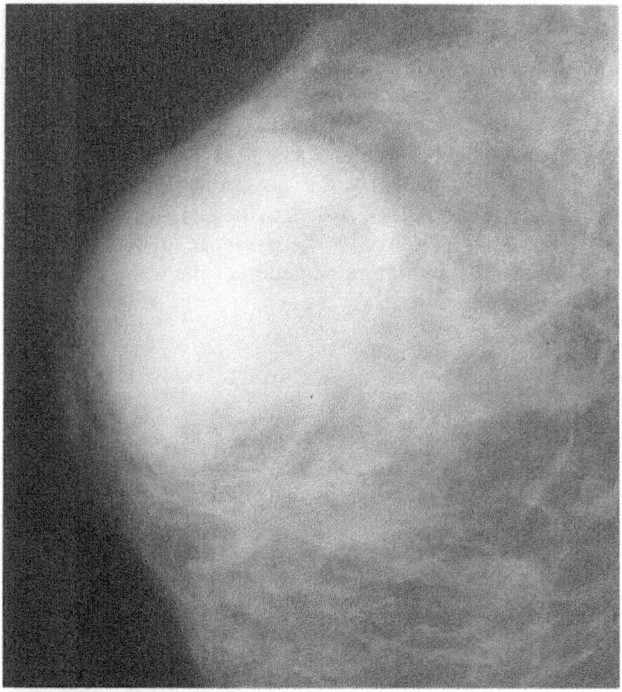

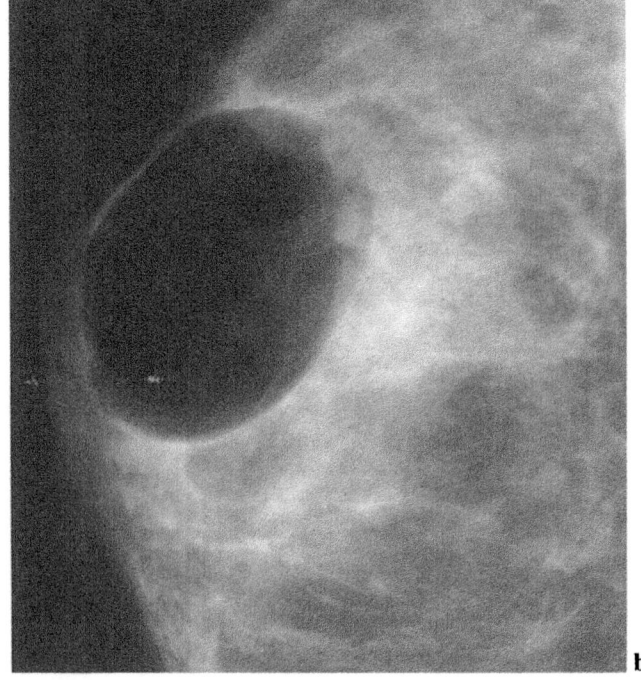

a

b

Radiographs performed before (**a**) and after (**b**) puncture. In the transparent **36** breast note the huge opacity with a major axis of about 5 cm. On clinical investigation the nodule appeared to be well delineated, fluctuant, and elastic, suggesting a cyst. Ultrasonography of course, provided indisputable evidence. Nevertheless, the evidence from ultrasonography is not sufficient to dispense with performing puncture followed by air insufflation; as a matter of fact, it is not so much the intracystic vegetations (most often readily visible with ultrasonography) which risk going undetected as it is certain small calcifications, which are better visible with air contrast (see the chapter about calcifications).

The radiograph taken after puncture and air insufflation shows another irregular opacity at the upper pole of the opacity, relatively infiltrating and poorly defined; in this case, exeresis is called for.

37

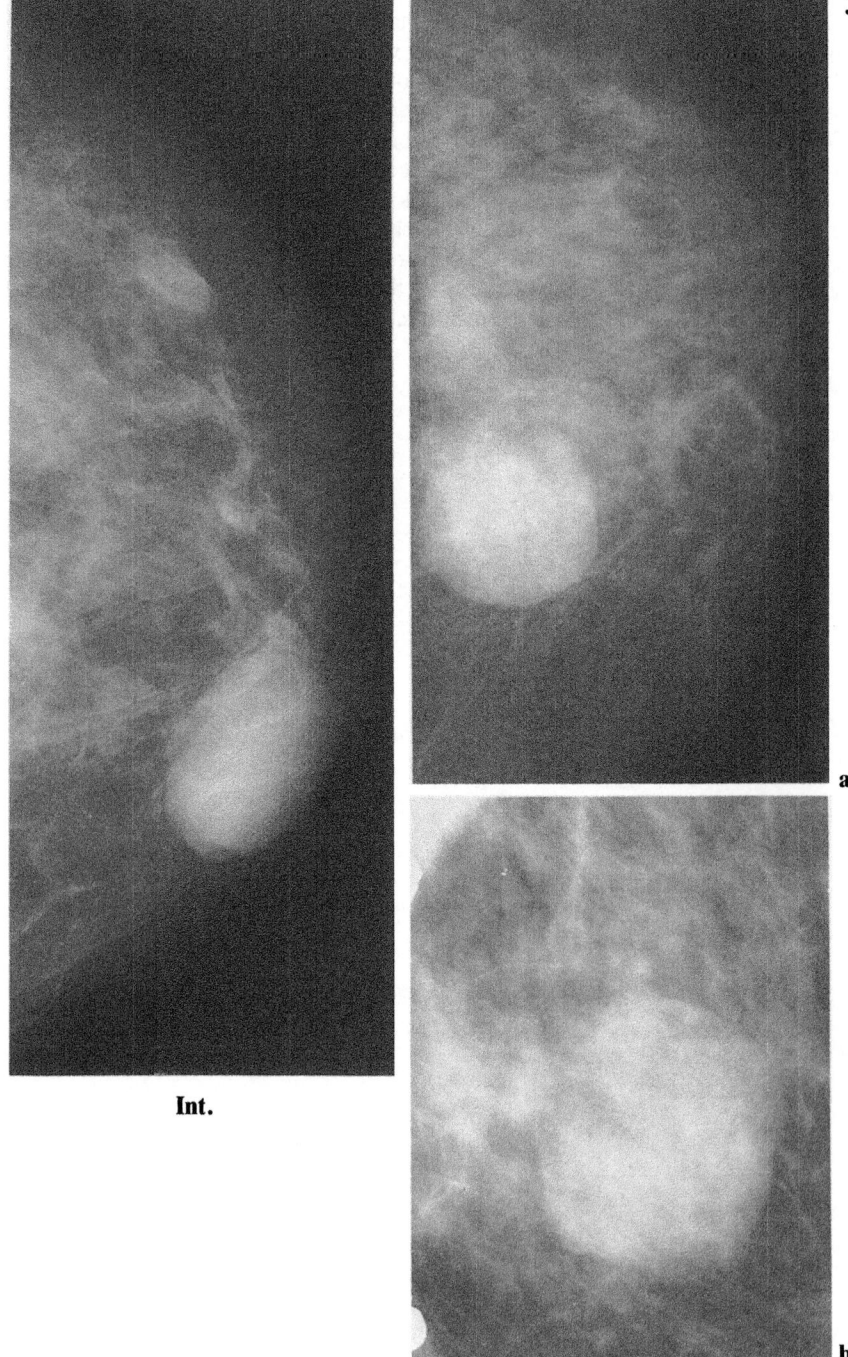

Int.

a

b

In the transparent breast several opacities are visible, a voluminous oval opacity, **37** situated in the medial left area, and a smaller one situated laterally. They are connected by marked vascular dilatation. Behind the smaller opacity, some other opacities are seen within a fibrotic patch. Needle biopsy of the medial nodule showed numerous carcinomatous cells, consistent with the diagnosis of a colloid-type epithelioma.

Since the lesions were diffuse, it was decided to perform a mammectomy. While the voluminous opacity in the medial area really corresponded to a colloid carcinoma, the smaller, lateral opacities were found to be consistent with fibrocystic mastopathy.

Fibrotic breast with multiple images of nodular fibrosis and a voluminous opacity **38** corresponding to a palpable nodule.

This huge opacity is dense, homogeneous, and rather well delineated on its medial aspect. In contrast, the lateral border has a halftone and blurred appearance (**a**).

The spot film shows the perfect regularity of almost the entire contour; on its anterior pole (lateral view) it is irregular and blurred, with infiltrations (**b**).

Needle biopsy showed the presence of numerous carcinomatous cells. The cytological diagnosis was a medullary epithelioma.

39

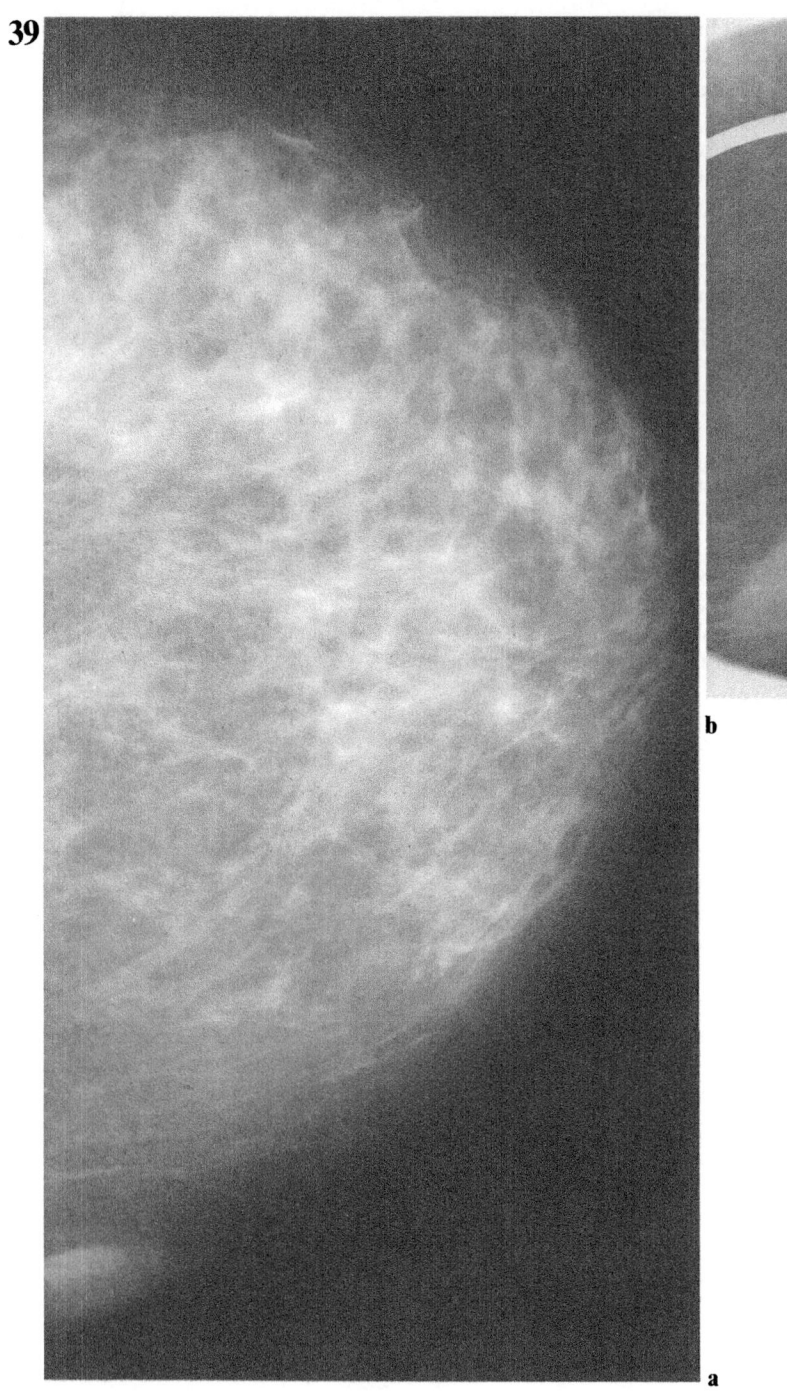

Int.

62

Normal breast; the only abnormality is an oval, subcutaneous opacity seen in the **39** very medial area (**a, b**), the site of which suggests a subcutaneous lesion. Based on the appearance and site of the opacity, a diagnosis of epidermal cyst was made. This was confirmed histologically. **a** Craniocaudal view, **b** detail of centre

40

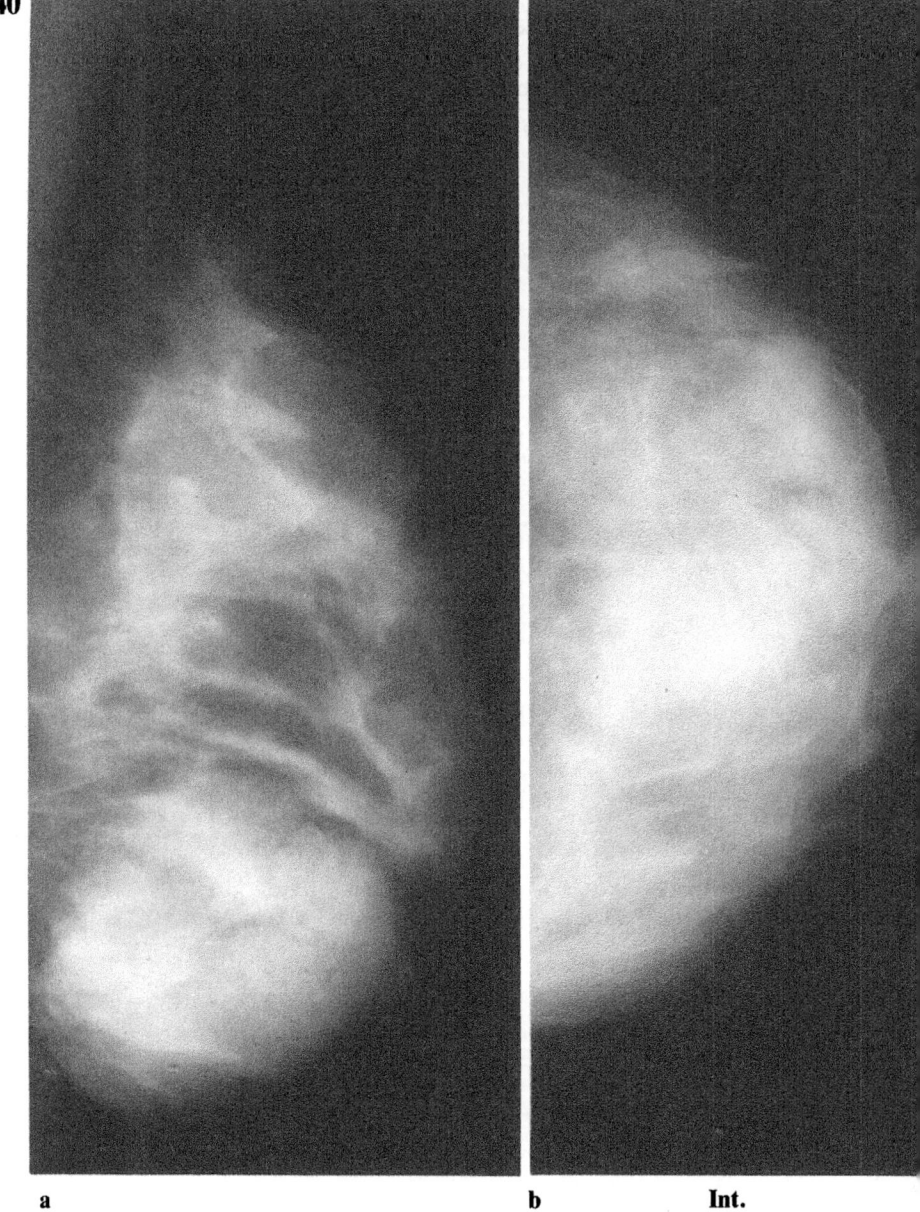

a   b   Int.

Right breast of a 21-year-old woman, treated homeopathically for a chronic **40** inflammatory syndrome for 3 years.

The radiological investigation (**a, b**) showed a large opacity which was rather homogeneous and well delineated, causing compression of the adjacent tissues. The case history and the appearance of the skin suggested the diagnosis of a chronic abscess, which was confirmed by surgery.

Abscesses of the breast in the acute inflammatory phase should be treated by surgical incision performed prior to antibiotic therapy, as the breast is a poorly vascularized organ which does not permit efficient concentration of antibiotics. Primary antibiotic therapy produces sedation of the acute inflammatory symptoms but leads, as in this case, to chronicity. Note that excision of this chronic mastitis required a true quadrantectomy. **a** Lateral view, **b** craniocaudal view

41
42

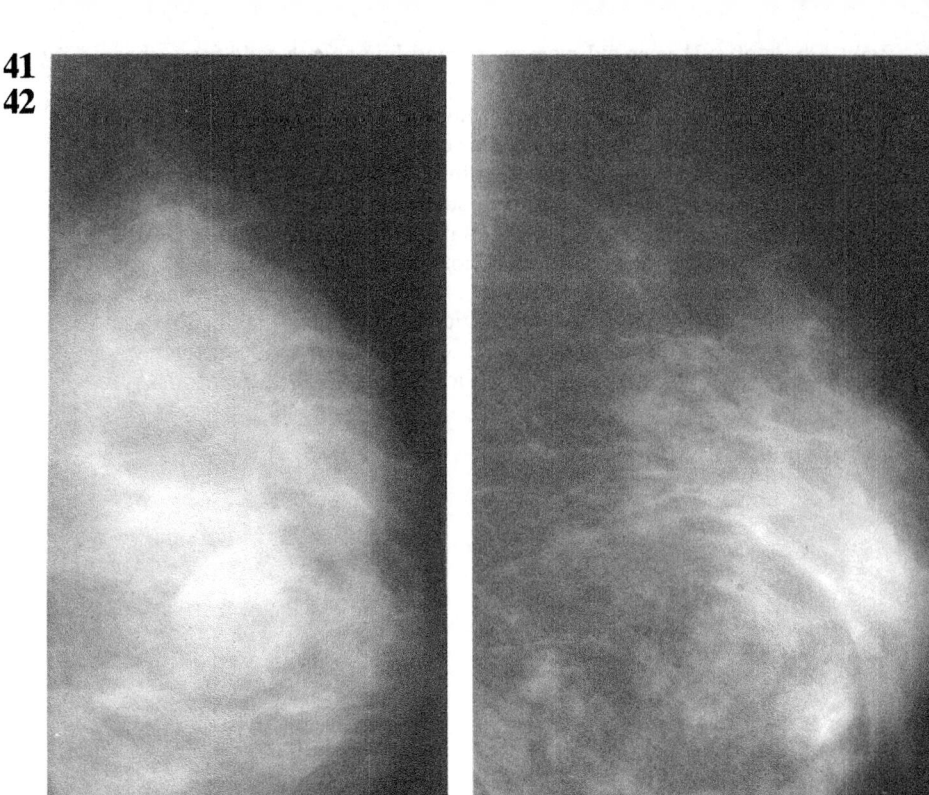

41

42

In the dense breast of a woman of 20, an opacity consistent with the presence of a **41** smooth and well-delineated nodule is seen; this is painful during the premenstrual period. The opacity is dense and homogeneous; it is poorly defined with regard to the adjacent tissues.

Cytology confirmed the diagnosis of a fibroadenoma. Fibroadenomas are often difficult to detect because of the high density of the breast in young women.

Ultrasonography is of great help in such cases; it shows a solid-type lacunar image without posterior attenuation.

Perfect image of an extended lipomatous translucency (7 cm in the major axis) **42** containing several smaller opacities that are heterogeneous and more or less rounded. This "breast-within-the-breast" appearance corresponds to that of a fibroadenolipoma (or a hamartoma).

43

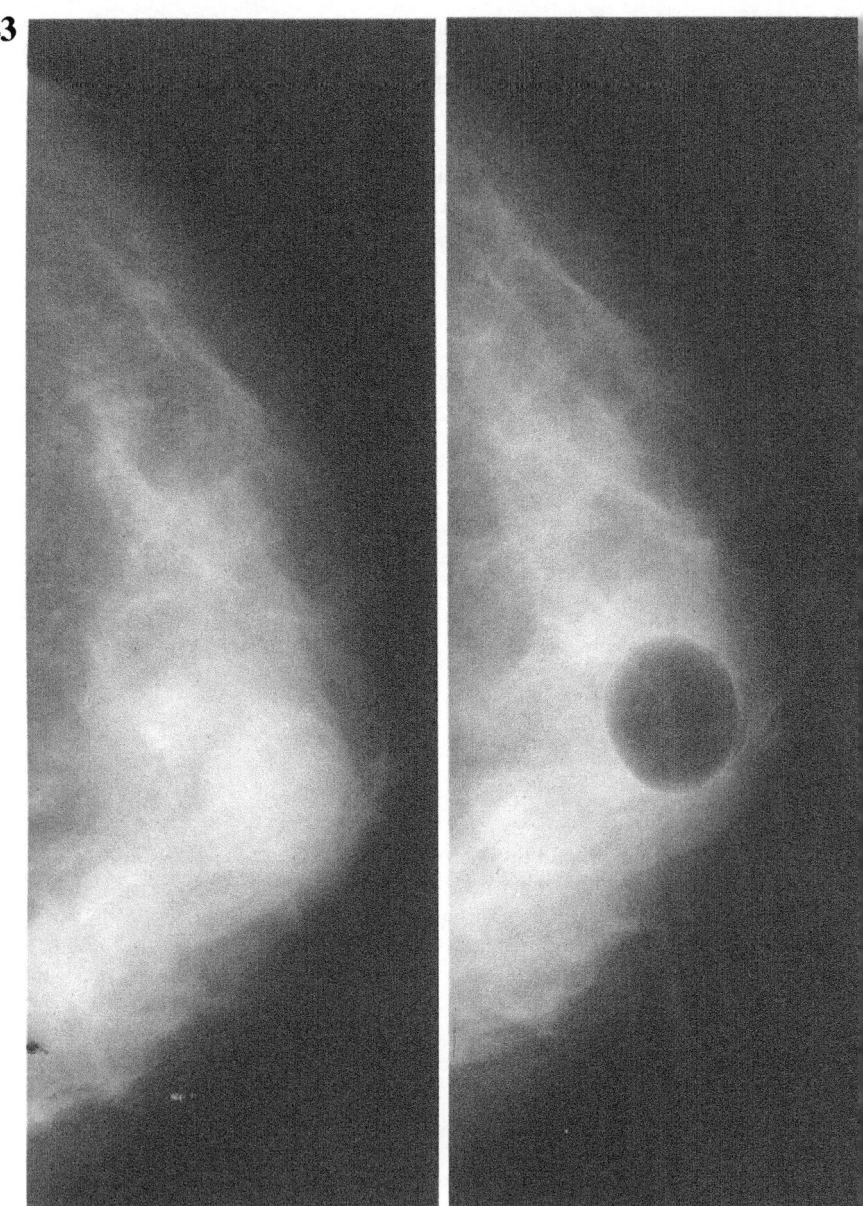

a   b

Radiographs made before (**a**) and after (**b**) puncture. A dense breast with two **43** opacities, one in the retromammilary area, the other slightly laterally. These opacities are dense, homogeneous, and relatively well delineated. Between them lies an opacity which is responsible for the blurred appearance of the posterior pole of the retromammilary opacity (*1*).

This case illustrates perfectly the fact that information provided by ultrasonography is not always sufficient. As a matter of fact, ultrasonography showed the absence of intracystic vegetations, and only puncture with air insufflation showed the intermediate opacity to be a superimposition image, a benign cyst.

44

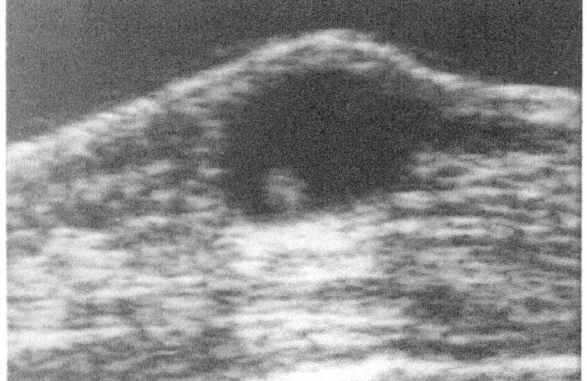

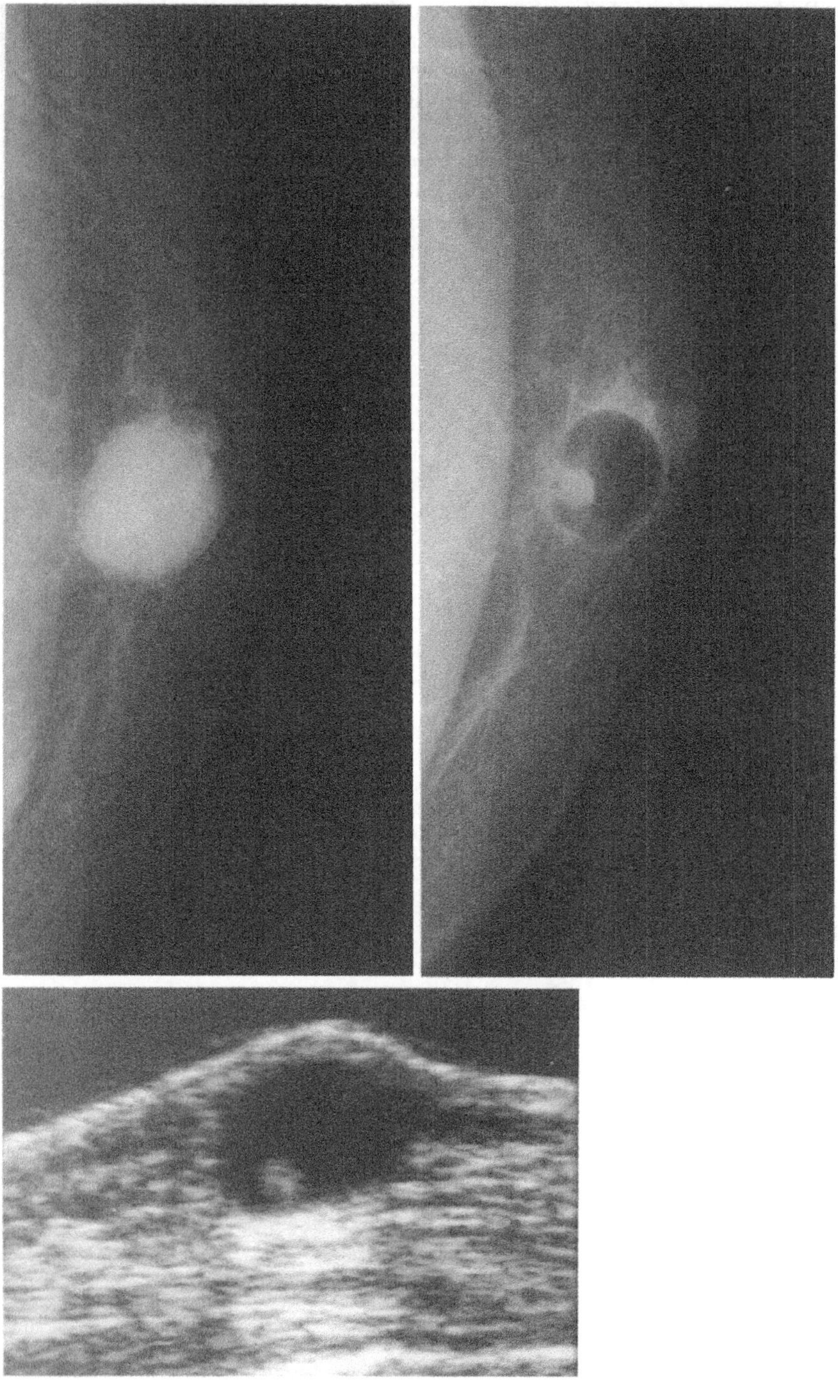

The male breast can be affected by the same pathology as the female: in this case, **44** a cyst is seen, prior to (**a**) and after (**b**) puncture.

The plain film (**a**) shows a dense, homogeneous opacity which is well delineated; at the level of its medial aspect is a small opacity corresponding to the nipple, which is not tangential.

Ultrasonography (**c**) shows indisputably the image of a liquid cyst with an intracystic vegetation. Air insufflation permits perfect visualization, not only of the vegetation but also of its insertion.

Radiography never confirms whether these vegetations are benign or malignant, so excision is indispensable in any case.

Histology showed a benign dendritic vegetation.

45

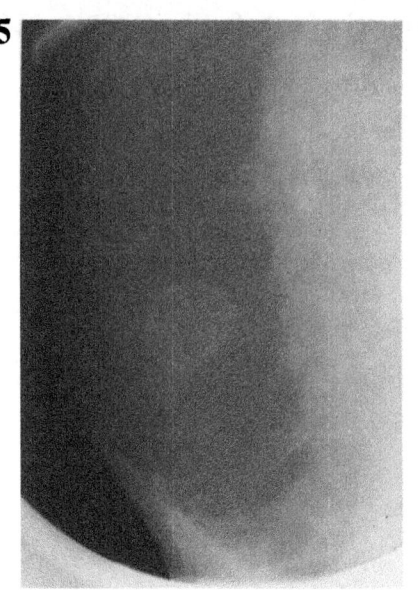

46

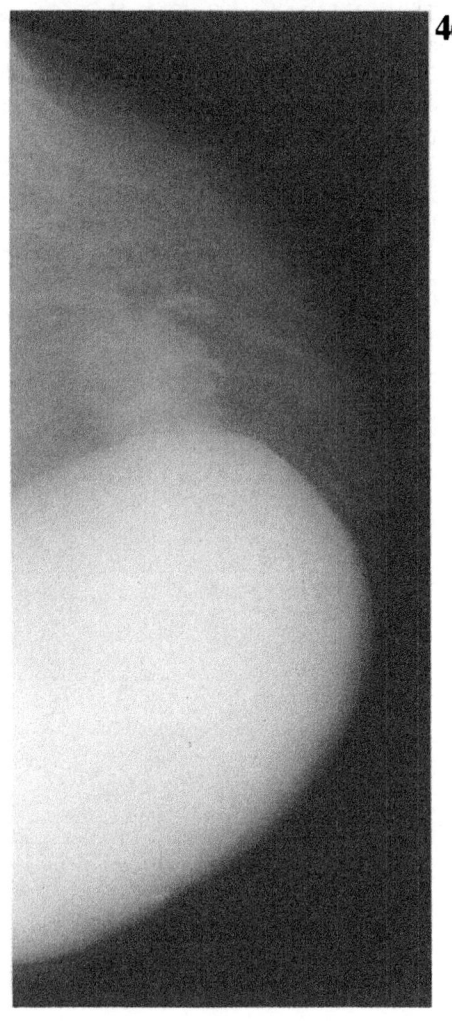

After a severe trauma to the right breast, a hard nodule has appeared. The **45** radiograph shows a very thin, rounded opacity surrounding a clear image. This is the typical appearance of steatonecrosis, which can later on become responsible for parietal calcifications (see *Microcalcifications*).

A 50-year-old woman was examined because of a rapidly growing mass. **46** Development of the tumor was so fast that it had caused marked cutaneous lesions (redness and thinning of the skin, preulcerative appearance).

Thermography shows hyperthermia, and radiographic investigations show a dense, homogeneous opacity, comparable to the opacity of fibroadenoma. The clinical data (explosive growth) suggested the diagnosis of phyllode tumor; histology confirmed this diagnosis.

Note, also in the medial area, the presence of another rounded opacity, much less dense, very likely corresponding to another phyllode tumor at an early stage of development.

47

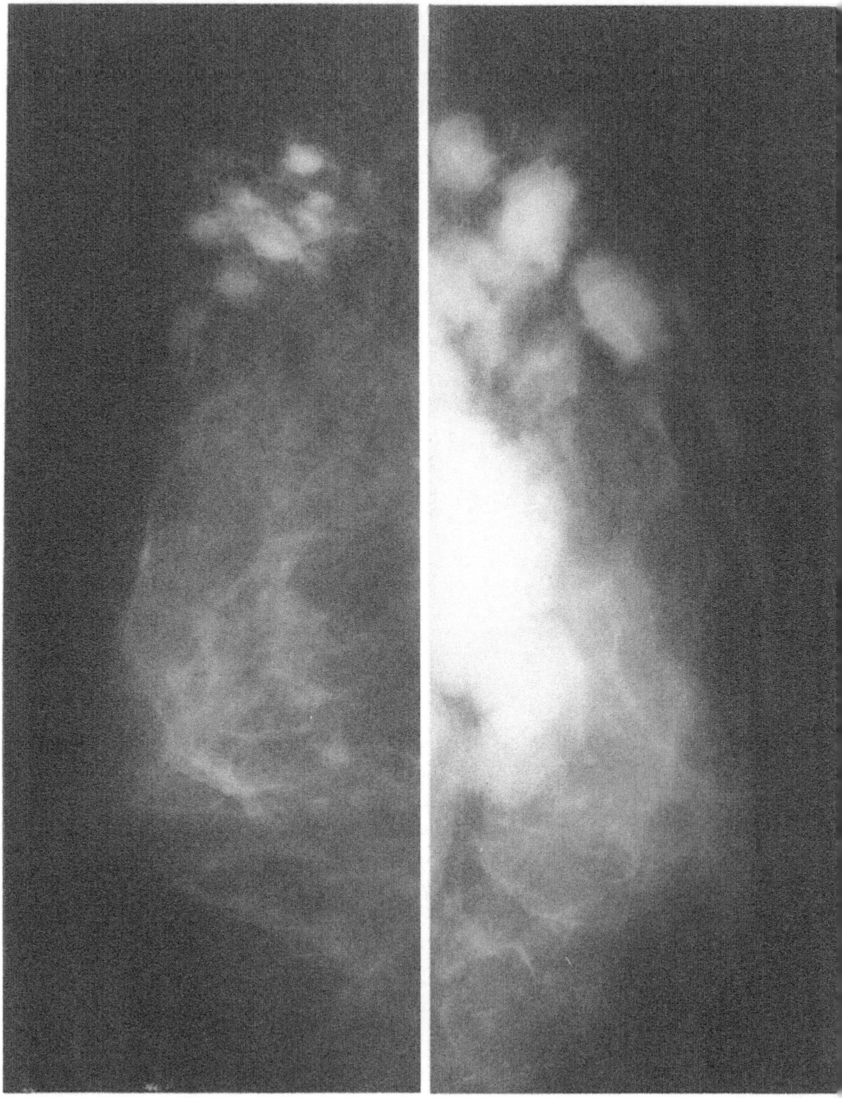

The breast (**a, b**) of a patient who had undergone plastic surgery 15 years earlier (silicone protheses). There is fragmentation of the prosthetic material, with migration of silicon fragments as far as to the subclavicular area.

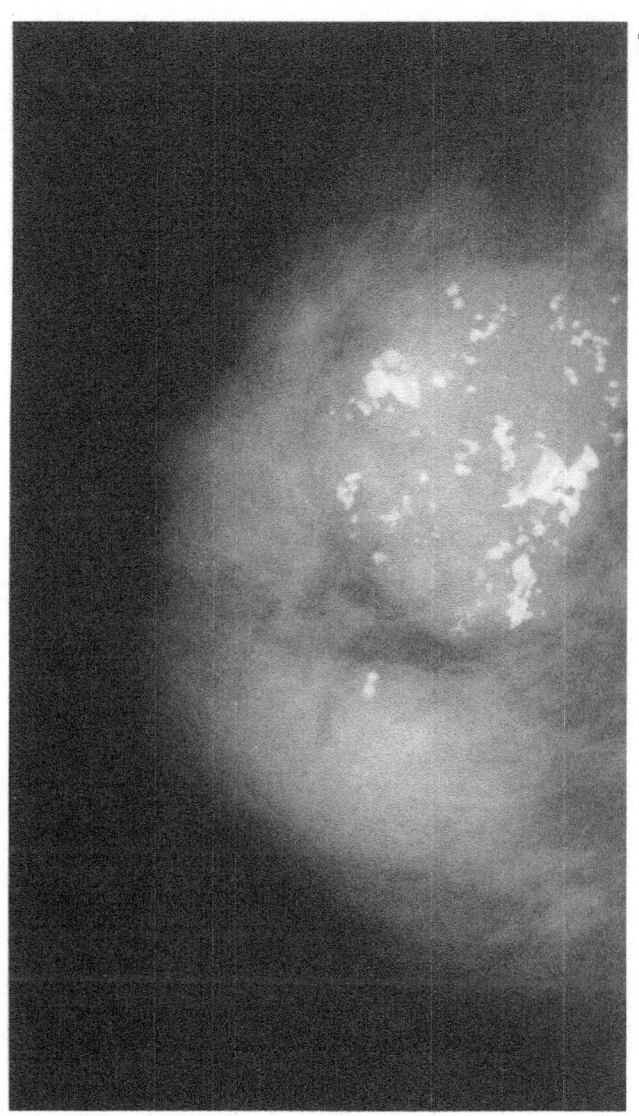

48

A voluminous, dense, homogeneous, and well-outlined opacity is seen in a very dense breast with numerous fibrotic patches, especially in the lower area.

The thick, dense and ribboned calcifications progressively surrounding the opacity suggest the diagnosis of a fibroadenoma undergoing calcification.

49

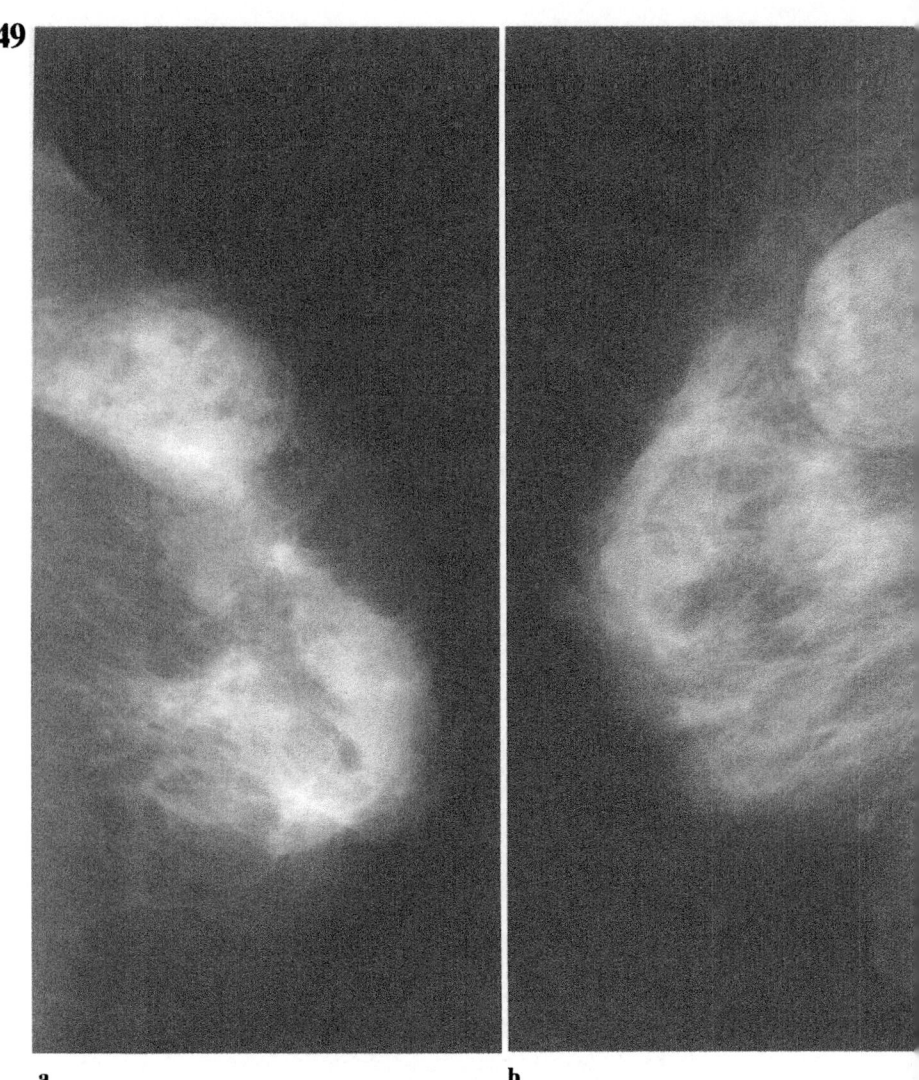

a   b

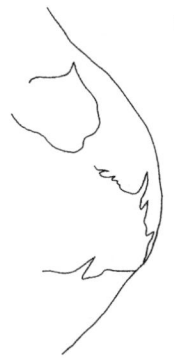

Superolateral, relatively heterogeneous opacity with smooth contours in a dense breast.

On the frontal view (**a**), note the fibrous expansion corresponding to a Duret's crest (see schemata). The lateral view (**b**) decomposes the fibrous crests and shows an anterior linear opacity in front of the first opacity.

The latter corresponds to a patch of fibrosis, as suggested by its perfectly smooth contour.

50

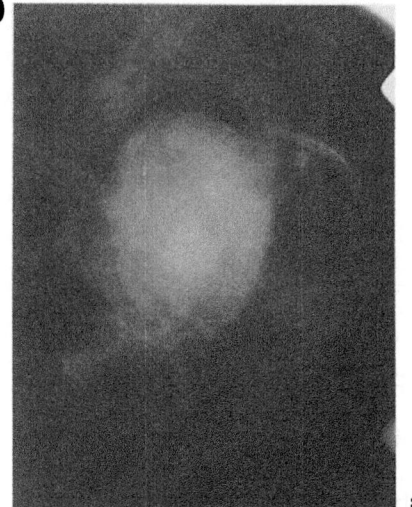

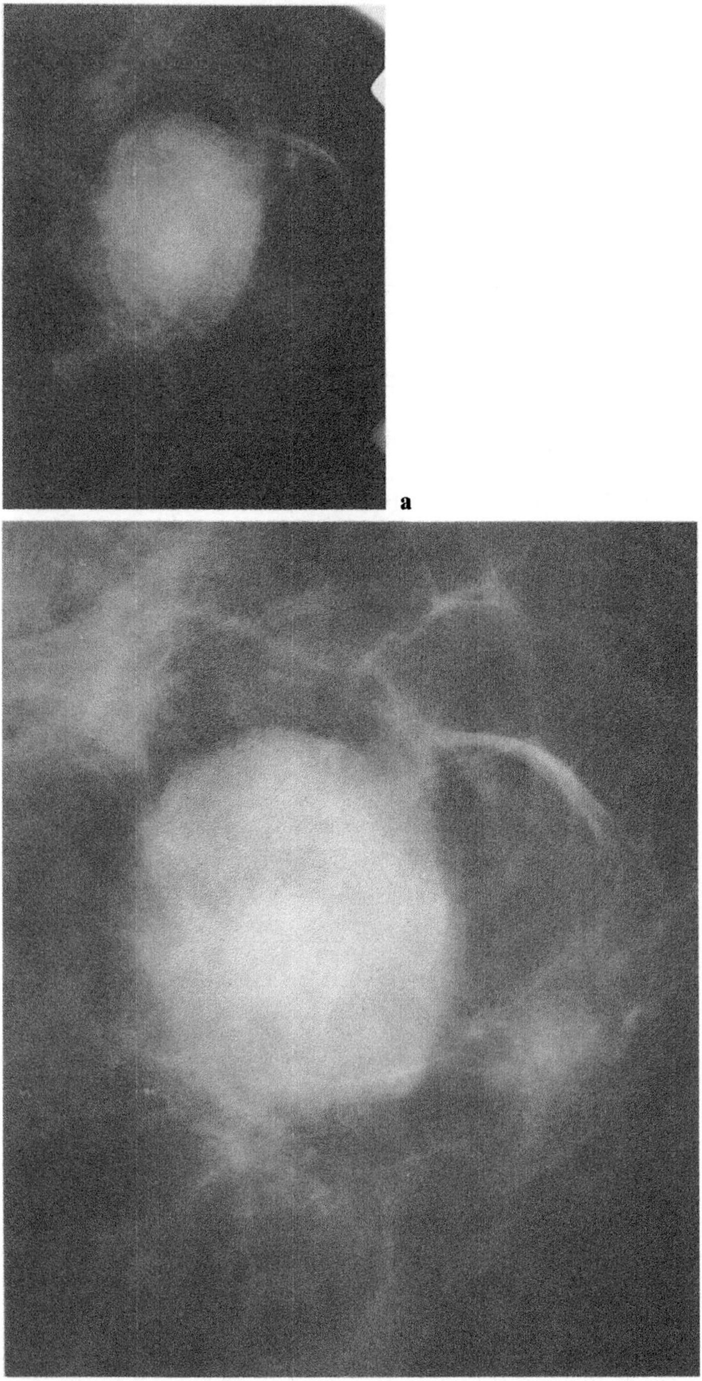

a

b

Dense, homogeneous, and well-delimited opacity in a postmenopausal breast **50** (a).

Careful study of the contours of the opacity shows, at the level of the posterior pole, rupture in the structural organization with a discrete expansion.

The diagnosis of cancer must be considered: the image of the opacity, shown in detail with its comet-tail appearance on the magnified spot film (**b**), corresponds to a medullary carcinoma. Note the presence of heterogeneous, polymorphous calcifications, which are seen on the magnified spot film at the level of the posterior contour.

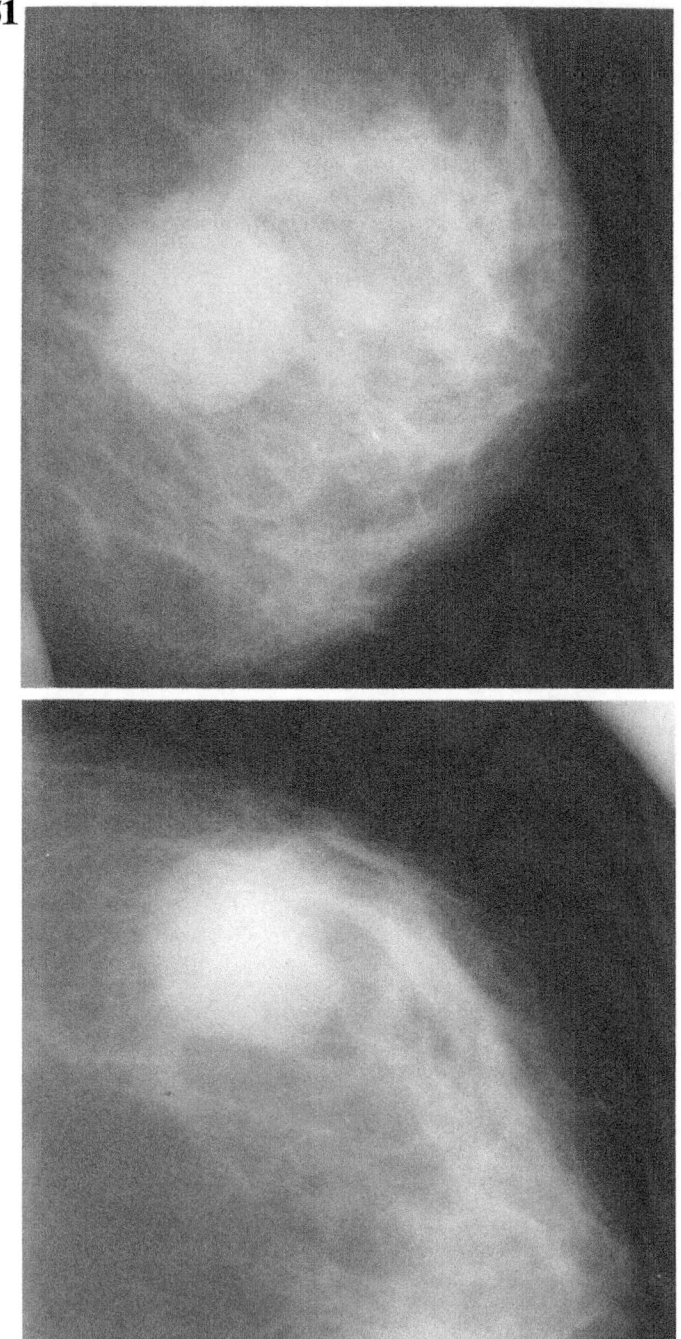

a

b

Dense, homogeneous and well-delineated opacity with a posterior expansion **51** (comet-tail) (**a, b**). Histology confirmed, in this case as well, the diagnosis of a medullary carcinoma.

Note the perfect regularity of almost the entire contour of the tumoral opacity.

52

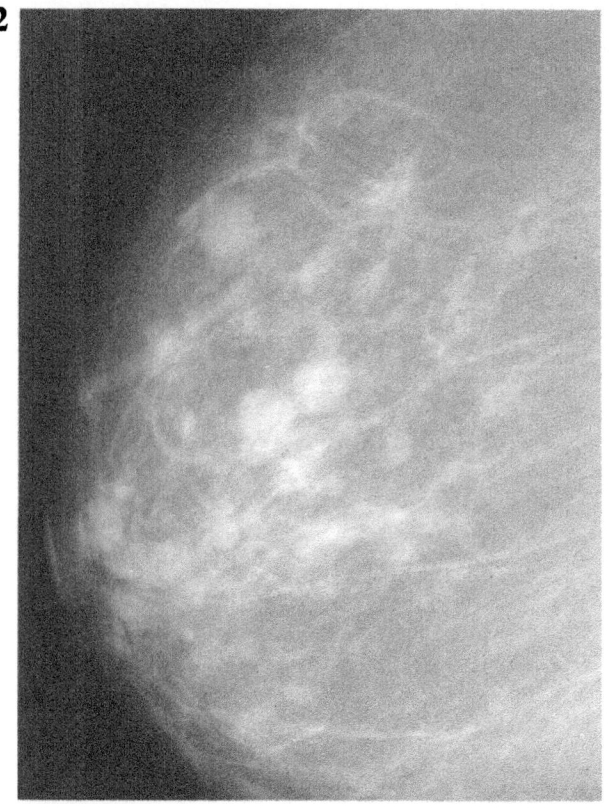

53

Postmenopausal breast with multiple dense and homogeneous opacities.   **52**
A careful analysis of the contour of each opacity shows that there is always at least one irregularity, i. e., expansion, or rupture in the structural organization. There are also multiple vascular calcifications, and a stellate opacity is seen in the upper area.

Histological investigation showed the existence of an invasive epithelioma (stellate image); the opacities correspond to cribriform epitheliomas.

The question may be asked, but histology hardly ever answers it: Could these opacities correspond to metastases from a carcinoma in the upper area of the breast?

This case illustrates one of the classical pitfalls associated with radiography of the **53** breast: A heterogeneous opacity with a few incisures is seen. It corresponds in fact to the projection onto the breast of a marked cutaneous tumor (hence, the advantage of constant radioclinical confrontation).

54

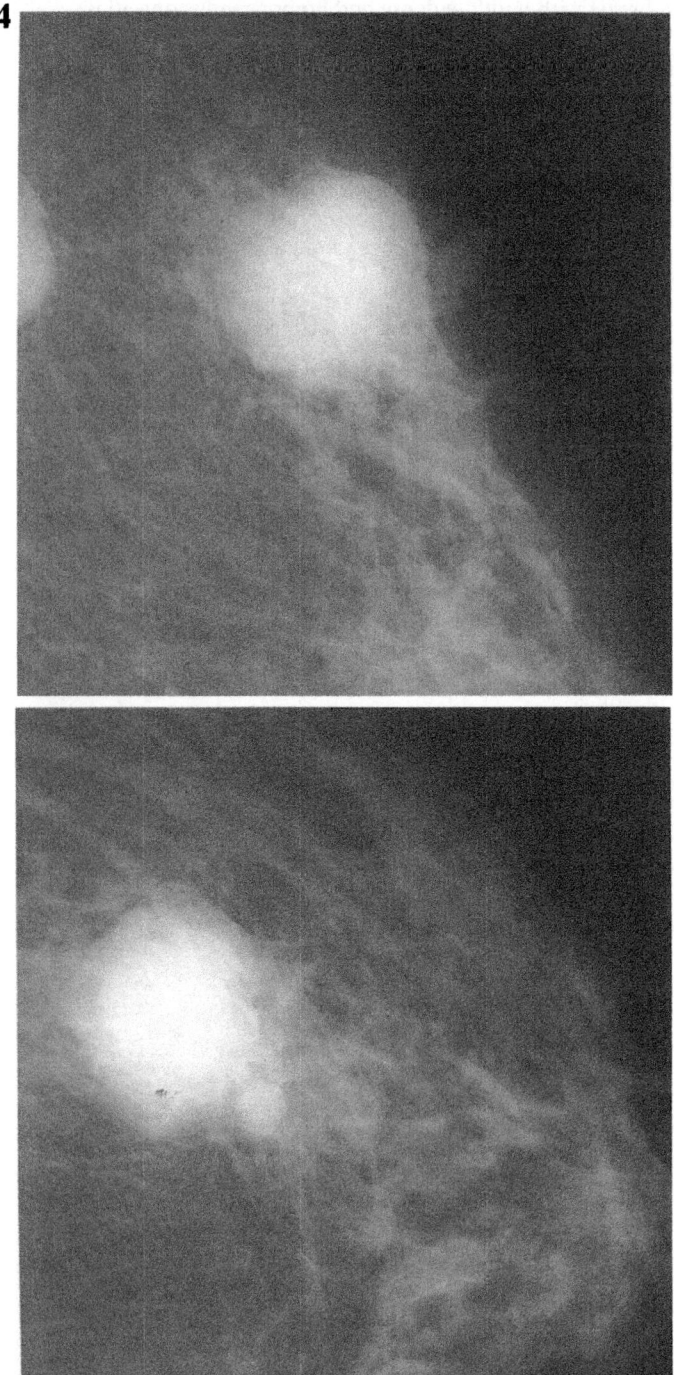

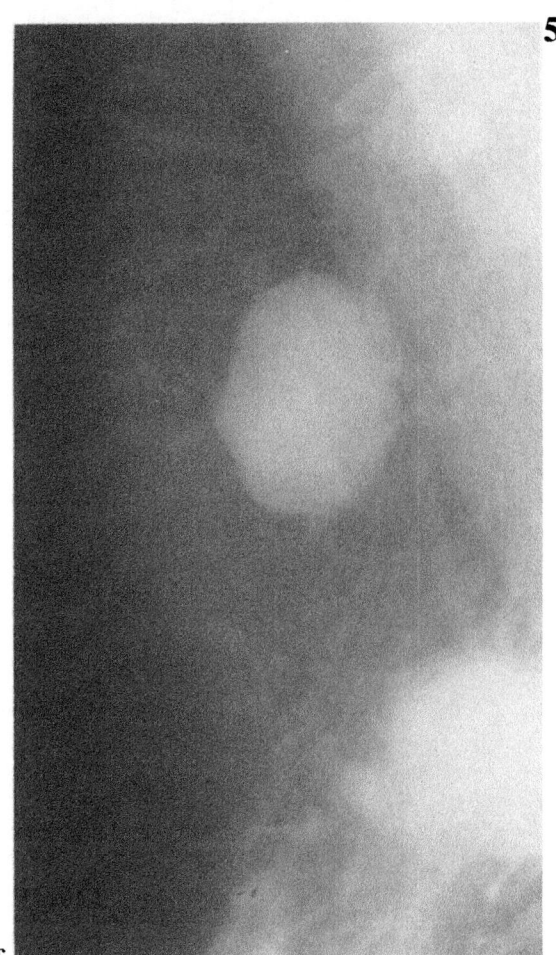

c

Dense, homogeneous opacity with multiple irregularities in the contour in a relatively clear and translucent breast. The radiologic appearance suggests a malignant lesion (**a, b**).

This case is of interest because of the detection in the axillary tail (**c**) of two lymph-node opacities, which are obviously neoplastic.

Radiographic investigations never reveal the nature of a node. Only elements of probability (marked increase in volume with presence of a carcinoma in the breast; irregular, spiculated appearance) usually permit one to consider the diagnosis of a lymph-node metastasis.

V. Microcalcifications

Calcifications measuring 0.1–0.5 mm in diameter have long been synonymous with carcinoma.

Improved techniques and increased knowledge of dysplasia have permitted a better definition of the malignancy criteria of these calcifications.

All classifications proposed to date have become less and less useful, since advances in technique and detection permit the visualization of ever smaller calcification foci with very few elements.

Existing classifications are accurate when they concern a large number of calcifications. For detection investigations they are practically of no interest.

Early diagnosis of breast cancer is in fact based on the analysis of elementary images:
- Calcifications
- Diffuse or localized opacities
- Changes in the structural organization of breast tissue
- Indirect signs

These images are encountered with carcinomas as well as with benign mastopathies. When considered suspect, their interpretation should take into account not only their morphological features but also their surroundings and their association.

As concerns noninfiltrating intraductal carcinomas, calcifications should be interpreted with regard to six criteria:
1. Size
2. Number
3. Location
4. Orientation
5. Density
6. Shape

Size: Calcifications in intraductal carcinoma in situ show great variations in size. They range from 0.1 mm to 0.5 mm, and are sometimes at the limit of visibility. This heterogeneity is certainly a feature which arouses suspicion.

Number: The first authors described "uncountable calcifications" in intraductal carcinoma in situ. A large number of calcifications is a definite indication for exeresis. As a rule, any group of more than four calcifications should be excised, when there are other suspicious patterns.

Location: Calcifications are diffuse and may involve a large area of the breast or be located in a small area. More important than location, however, is the shape of the projection area. Lanyi shows that geometrical projection figures very often correspond to carcinoma.

Orientation: In intraductal carcinomas, the calcifications are always orientated anarchically in all planes. They do not have a regular appearance as in dysplasia.

Density: The density is highly variable; some calcifications have the density of necrotic calcifications while others are hardly visible. Everything depends on the quality of the negative and on the speed at which the calcifications develop. Experience has also shown that, following exeresis of a specimen for biopsy, radiography shows a much higher number of calcifications in the parts operated.

Shape: This is certainly an indispensable aspect in diagnosing malignancy
- Rounded shape with a lighter center: necrotic calcifications.
- Rounded shape on the front-view negative, cupiliform on the side-view negative: calcifications in the fibrocystic state.
- Regular, linear calcifications: calcifications in certain inflammatory complaints.
- Rounded calcifications: lobular-type calcifications.
- Irregular, hook-shaped, V-shaped and vermicular: calcifications of intra-canalicular cancer.

Each of the characteristics discussed for the study of these calcifications permits a diagnosis that would point to a suspected carcinoma. Certainty in the diagnosis of malignity results from the concordance of the criteria described. Only when the heterogeneity in size, number, location, orientation, density, and shape of the calcifications has been ascertained is it possible to conclude the existence of carcinoma.

55

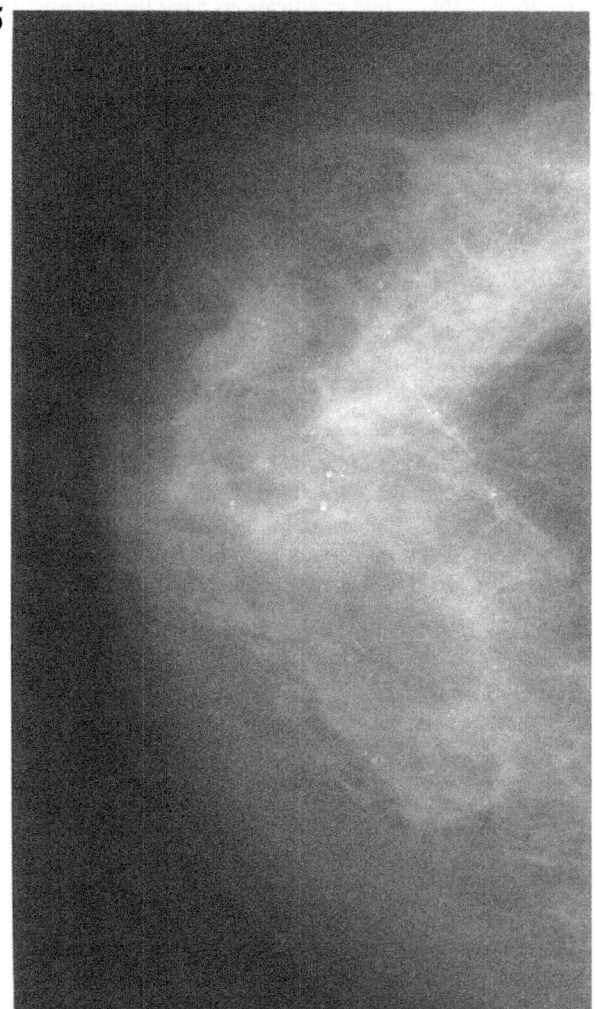

Int.

a

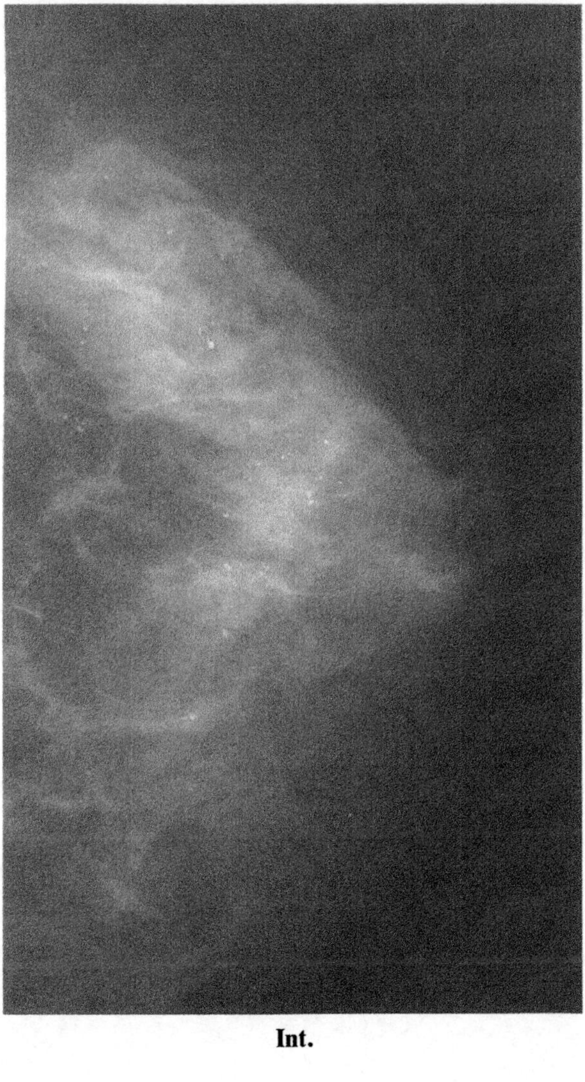

Int.

Frontal views, right (**a**) and left (**b**), of a dense breast with lateral patches of fibrosis, recognizable by their rectilinear margin. The visualized calcifications are diffuse, bilateral, and of rather unequal size; their density and shape are homogeneous.

These rounded, relatively regular calcifications correspond to calcifications often seen with dysplastic or hyperplastic lesions (adenosis).

Since they are diffuse, exeresis does not seem indicated because of the severe mutilation which would result, but since they are an undisputable risk factor, regular follow-up is advised.

56

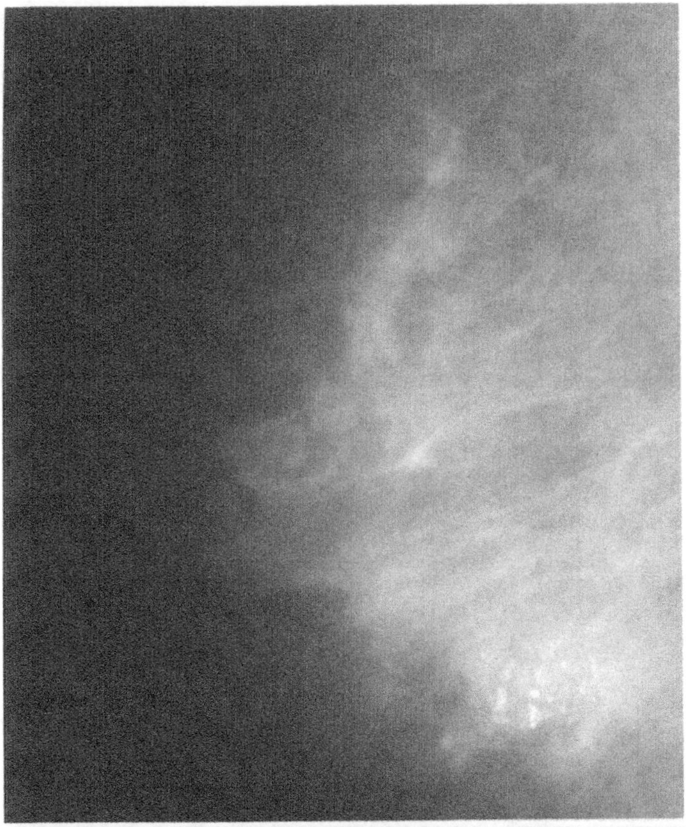

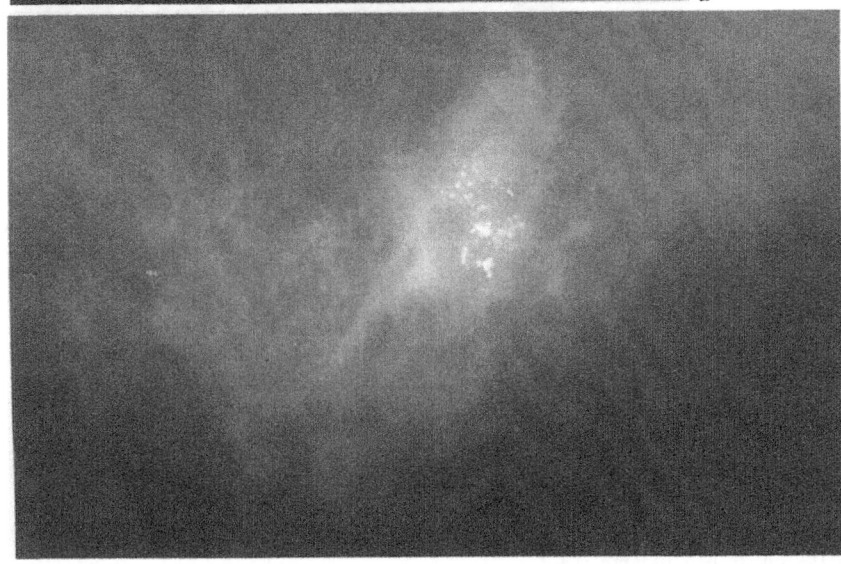

a

A small cluster of calcifications within a fibrous opacity (**a, b**). The calcifications **56** correspond in this case to five of the criteria of malignity listed above.

Excision was indispensable; it revealed a localized intraductal carcinoma, but the histological investigation showed microinvasion.

The microinvasion was predictable from the radiographs, which showed a dense and relatively irregular opacity surrounding the calcifications.

57

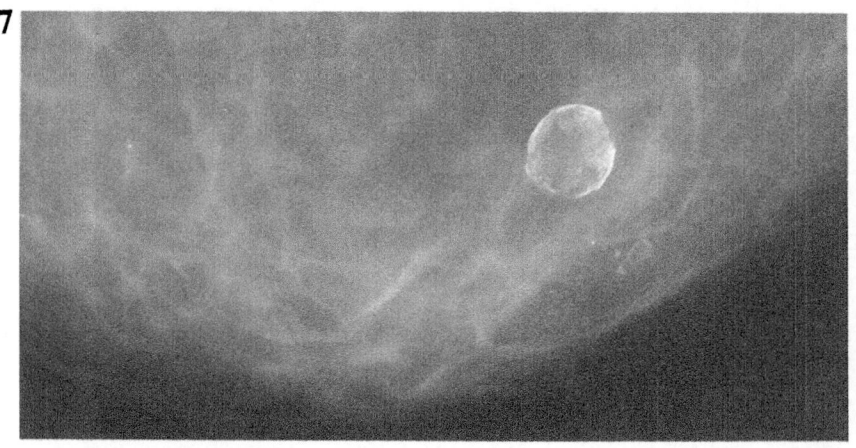

58

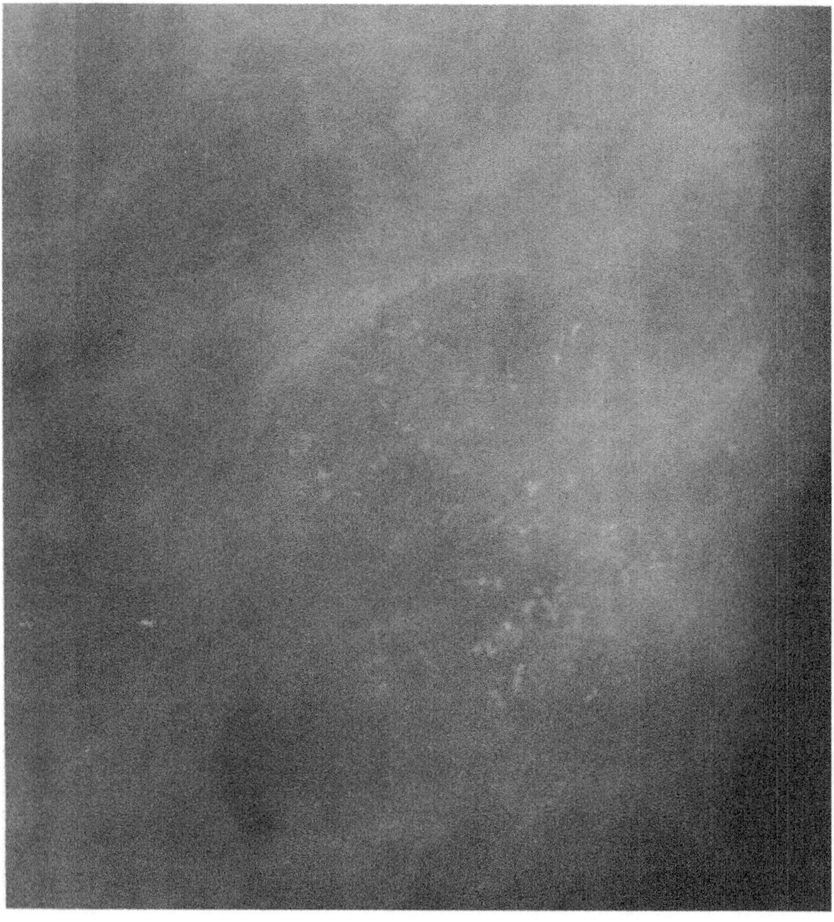

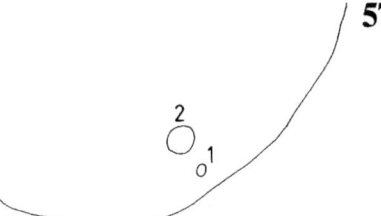

This case illustrates two different stages in the development of post-traumatic fat necrosis: The ultimate effect of such fat necrosis (*1*) is calcification (*2*). The calcifications are frequently seen during routine examinations.

Their consistent characteristic is a clear center. Besides in traumas, these images are seen after limited surgery and following repeated microtraumas (from, e. g., straps and underwiring in a brassiere). Cytosteatonecrosis calcifications should not be confused with the very fine and much smaller calcifications occurring in talcgranulomas (resorption granuloma).

Polymorphous calcifications, diffusedly and anarchically distributed, of unequal **58** density; diffuse epithelioma with marked intraductal involvement. The calcifications seem very localized and well circumscribed; they do not overlap the periphery of the translucency which surrounds them, corresponding to what is commonly called the "clear halo".

The absence of stroma reaction suggests the presence of rapid-growth cancers.

59

a   b

Two cases with fibroadenoma at different phases of calcification. **59**

During an early stage (**a**), dense, homogeneous and ribboned calcifications develop at the periphery of the tumoral opacity. Afterwards, they tend to completely surround the opacity.

When the fibroadenoma is completely calcified (**b**) the clinical examination may reveal a suspect, very hard and often adherent mass. Radiographic investigation can serve to reassure the patient.

60

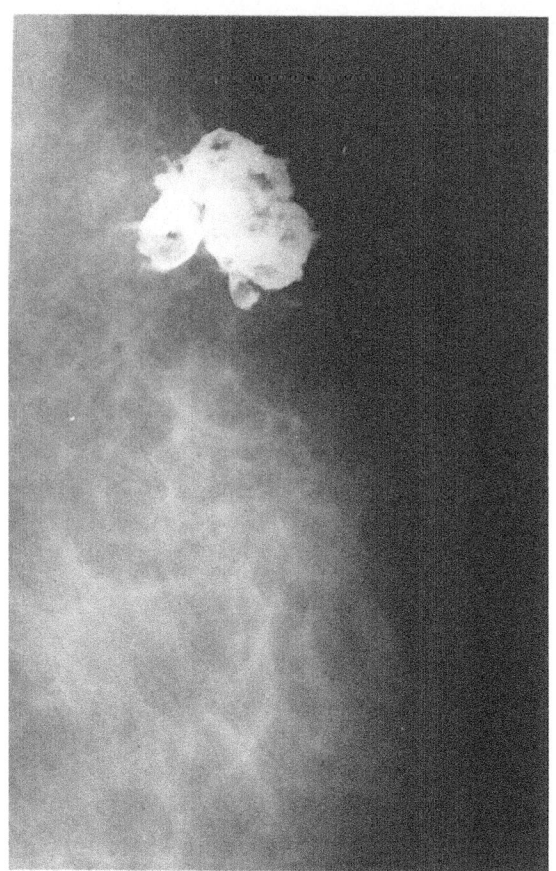

Bulky calcifications (with a clear center) in post-traumatic steatonecrosis. Trauma corresponds here to a scarring process following partial mastectomy and locoregional radiotherapy (superimpression focus with telecobalt 60).

This image is quite different from the previously shown calcifications in fibroadenomas. Note their clear center, which always allows correlation with an exogeneous cause.

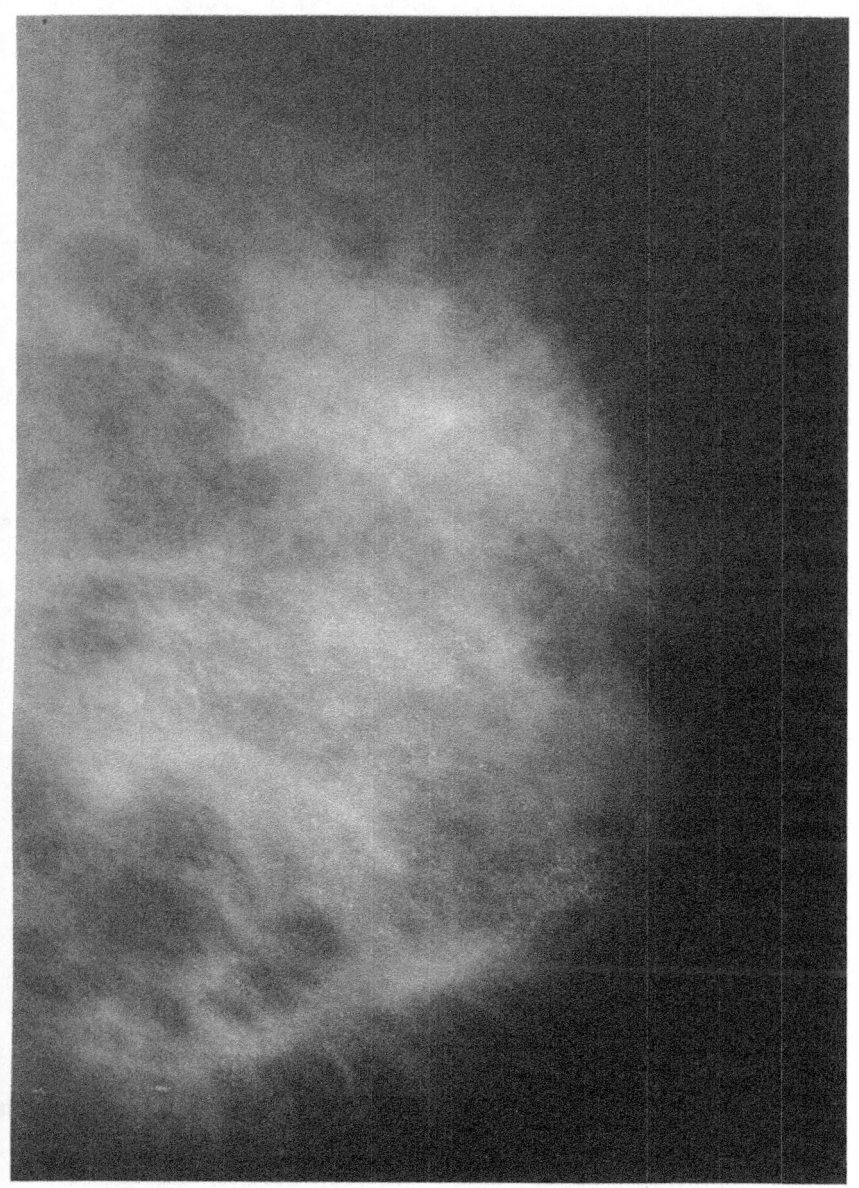

61

Diffuse calcifications throughout a breast with obvious signs of malignancy. Note the stroma reaction in the lower area, seen as linear, vertical opacities arising from a horizontal rupture in the structural organization. Histology revealed a highly evolutive and undifferentiated diffuse cancer.

62

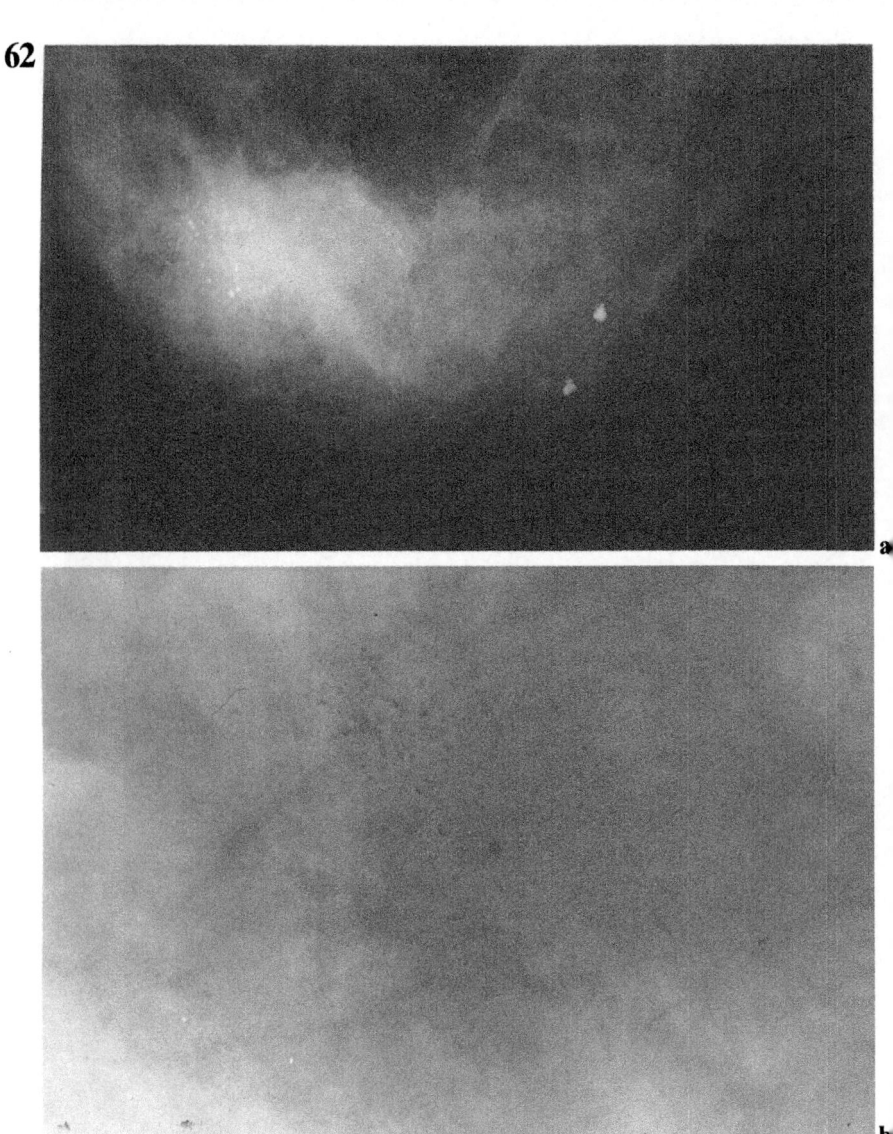

In the lateral part of the breast, diffuse calcifications corresponding to a diffuse **62**
epithelioma with intraductal involvement (**a, b**). The opacity shows signs of
ruptured architecture; one can thus conclude that the cancer is no longer
intraductal, but that there is already an invasive component.

Note the presence of benign bulky calcifications in the median area.

63

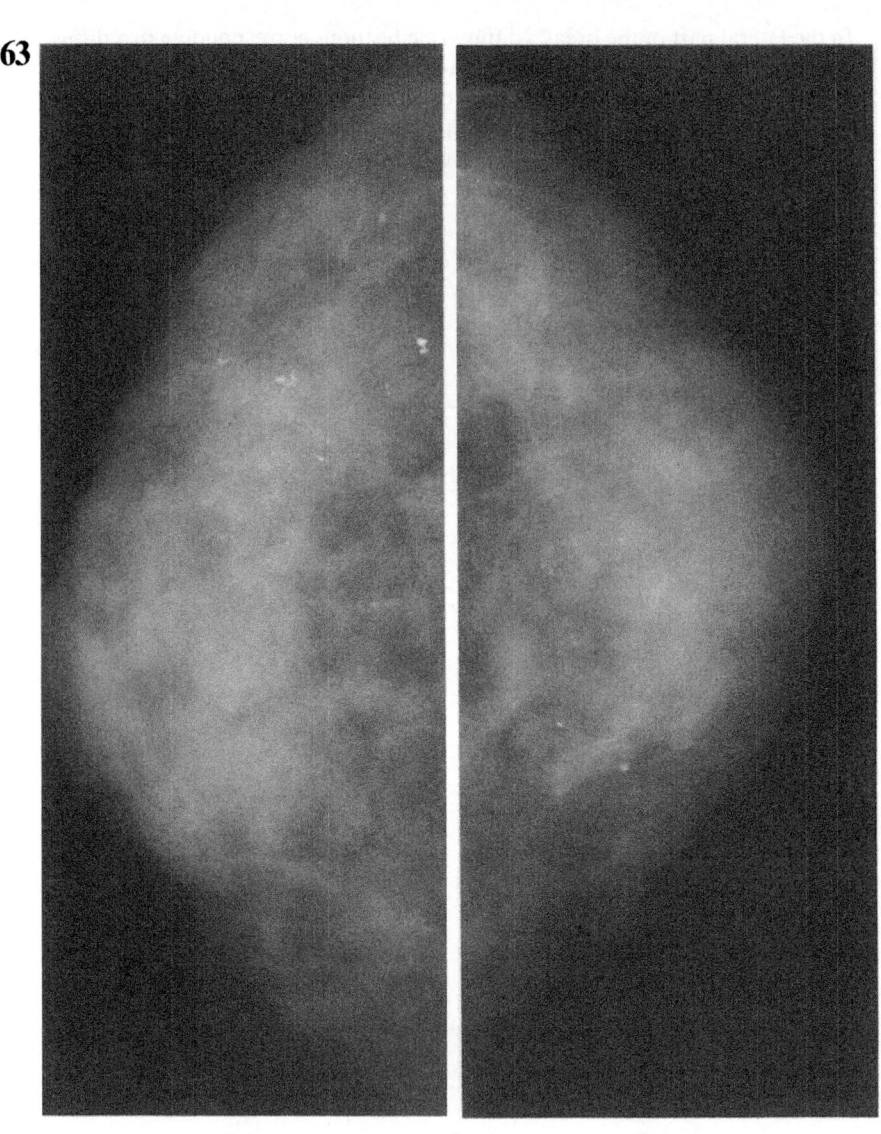

a   **Int.**   b   **Int.**

Bilateral calcifications; on the right (**a**) they are much more heterogeneous and occasionally form clusters, especially in the lateral area. Therapeutic strategy is difficult because of the bilaterality of the lesions; nevertheless, the appearance of the calcifications on the right is suspect enough to call for exeresis biopsy. Since this was done with the patient under general anesthesia, a contralateral biopsy was performed as well.

Histology showed a diffuse intracanalar, noninvasive epithelioma on the right (**a**), and on the left (**b**) an atypical lobular hyperplasia, which can be considered a borderline lesion.

Obviously, no definite diagnosis can be made from the radiographs.

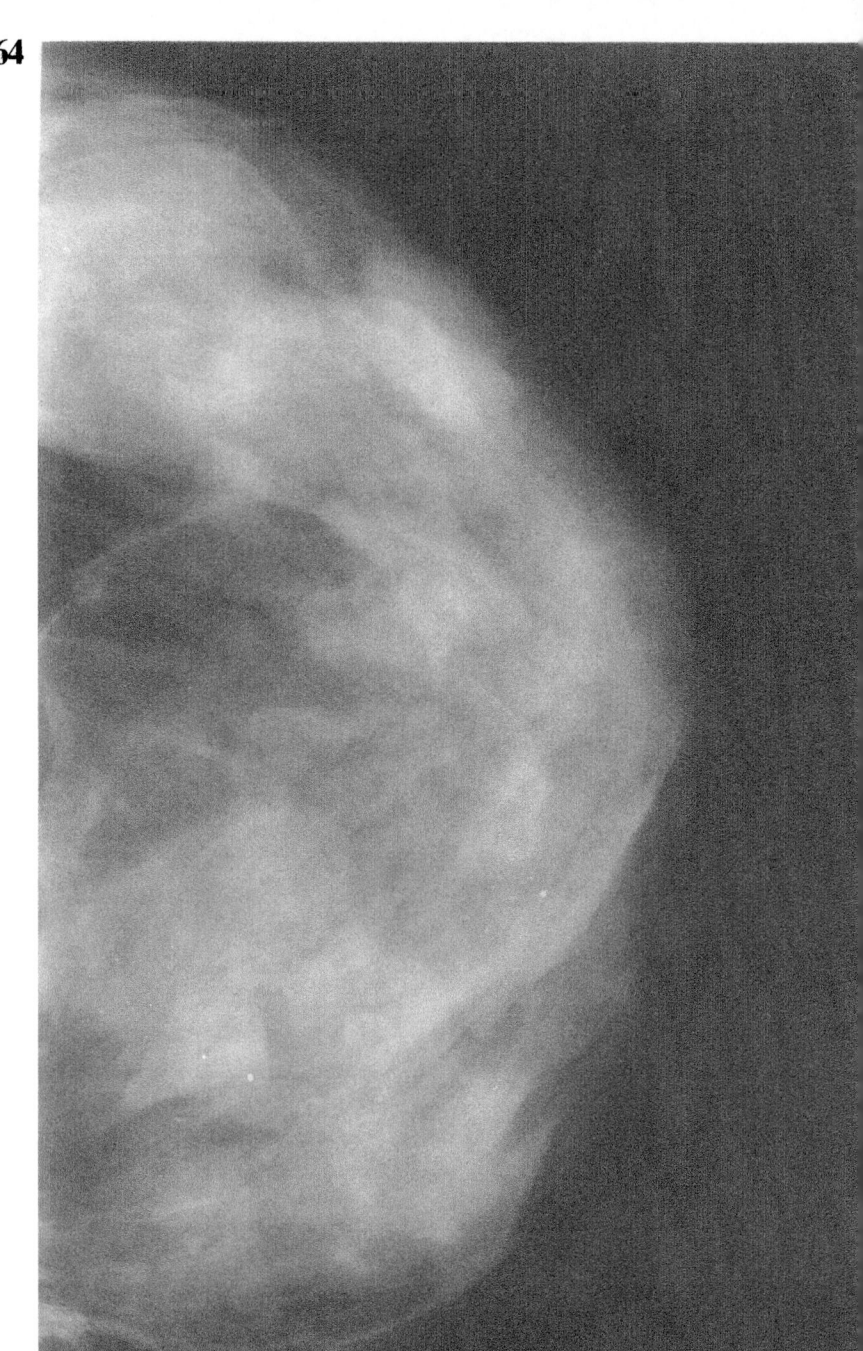

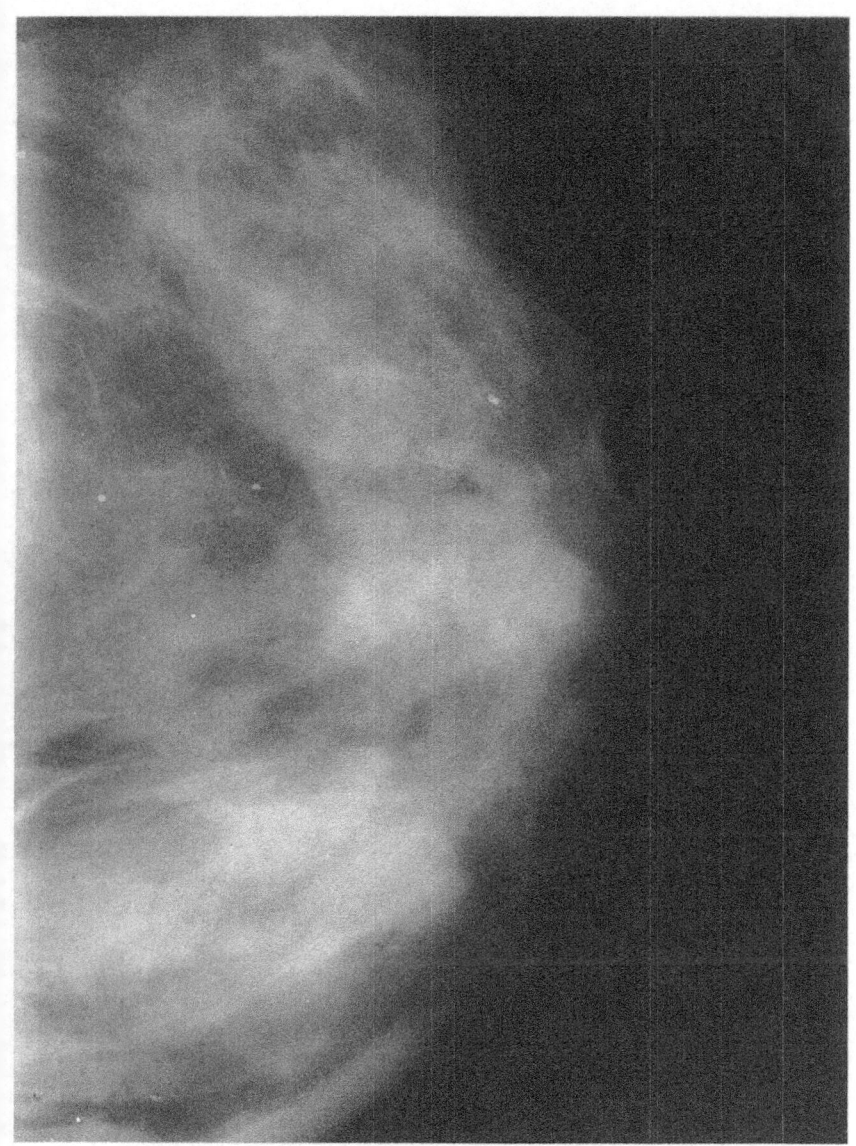

Ext.

b

Bilateral calcifications, most with a clear center, within a very homogeneously fibroglandular breast (**a, b**). The calcifications are quite benign; because they have a clear center they correspond to calcified cytosteatonecrosis.

Note the unusual and very rare appearance of linear fibrosis, especially in the lateral part of the right breast (**b**).

65

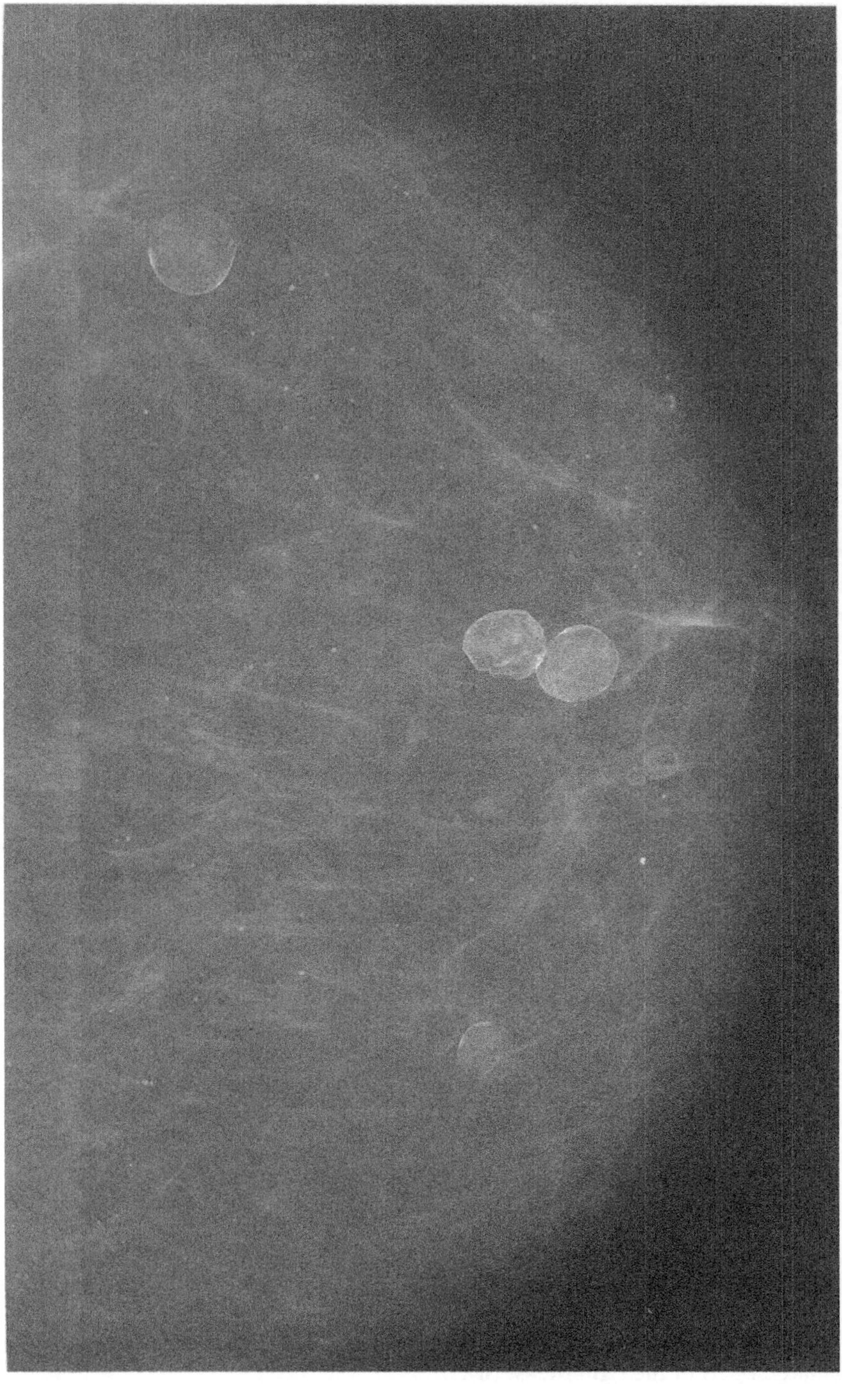

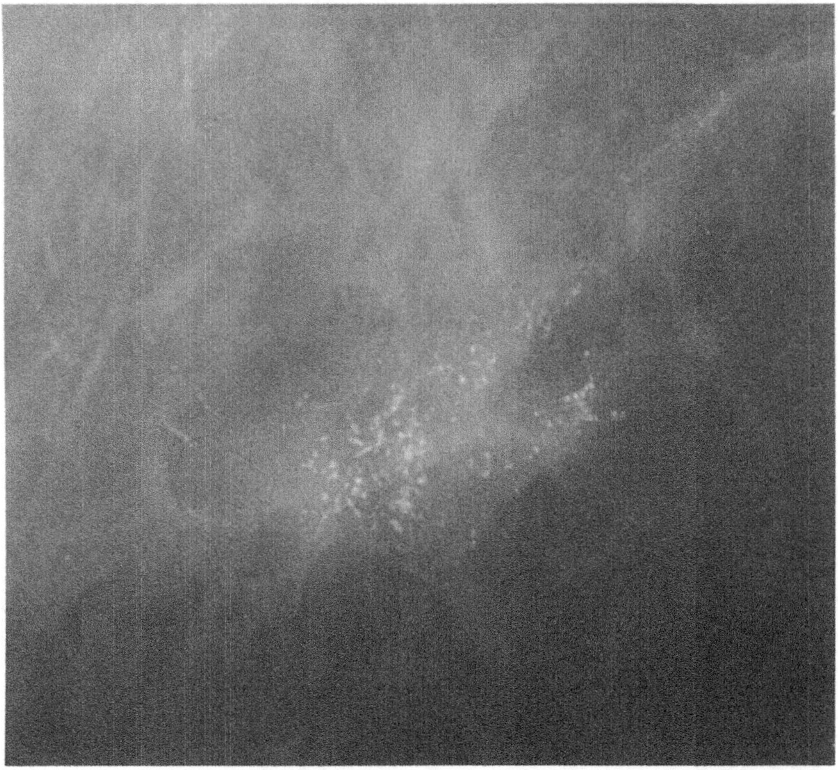

Perfect images of calcifications with clear centers corresponding to post-trau- **65**
matic fat necrosis. Note that these large calcifications, which correspond to
rupture in the structural organization of the retromammillary and are related to
anterior biopsy excision, are accompanied by a large number of small, rounded,
regular, and well-delineated calcifications.

These small calcifications are talcgranulomas (resorption granulomas).

This spot film shows not only highly polymorphous calcifications, heteroge- **66**
neously dense and arranged in clusters, but also an irregular opacity (structural
alteration); a diagnosis of malignancy is readily made.

Histological investigation showed an invasive epithelioma with marked
intraductal involvement.

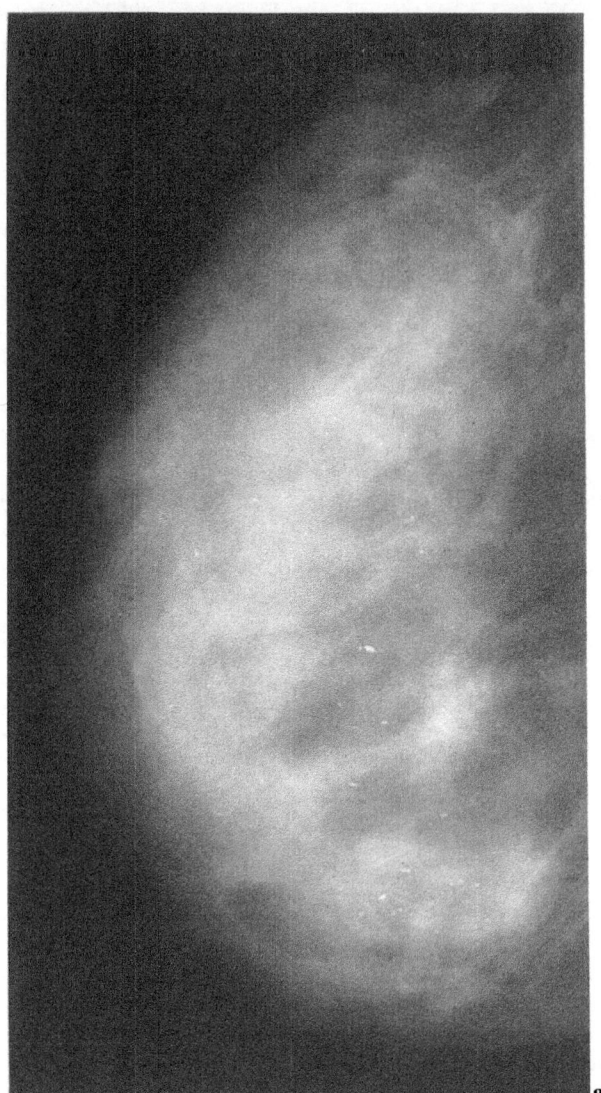

a

Both radiographs show regularly orientated calcifications, without polymorphism and of equal density. They are more numerous on the right side.

One should first of all search for a cluster of different calcifications. Grouping in clusters is one of the most reliable arguments for the diagnosis and the choice of treatment. In the present case, because of the appearance of the calcifications, simple follow-up was advised. The calcifications correspond indisputably to an atypical dysplastic lesion, to be considered a borderline pathology. These calcifications illustrate perfectly how inefficient are the classifications of microcalcifications proposed up to now.

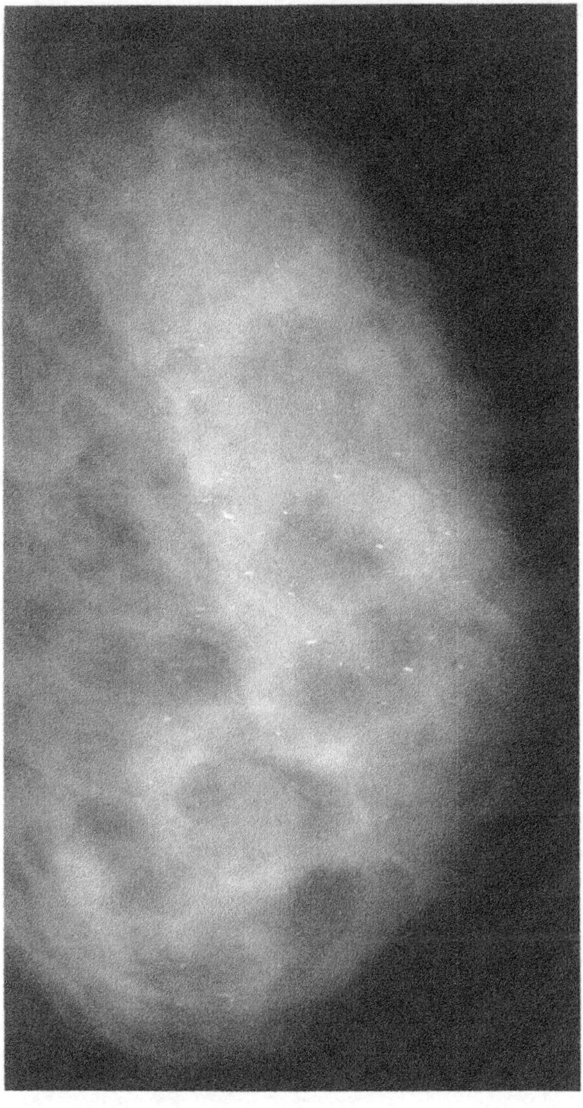

b

As a matter of fact, when the calcifications are very numerous, diagnosis poses no major difficulty.

The more frequent practice of high-risk exploratory investigation reveals the presence of few calcifications arranged in small clusters, which defy any classification. Excision must be based on signs provided by radiological investigation, on the radiologist's and the surgeon's experience, and possibly on the use of other techniques.

68

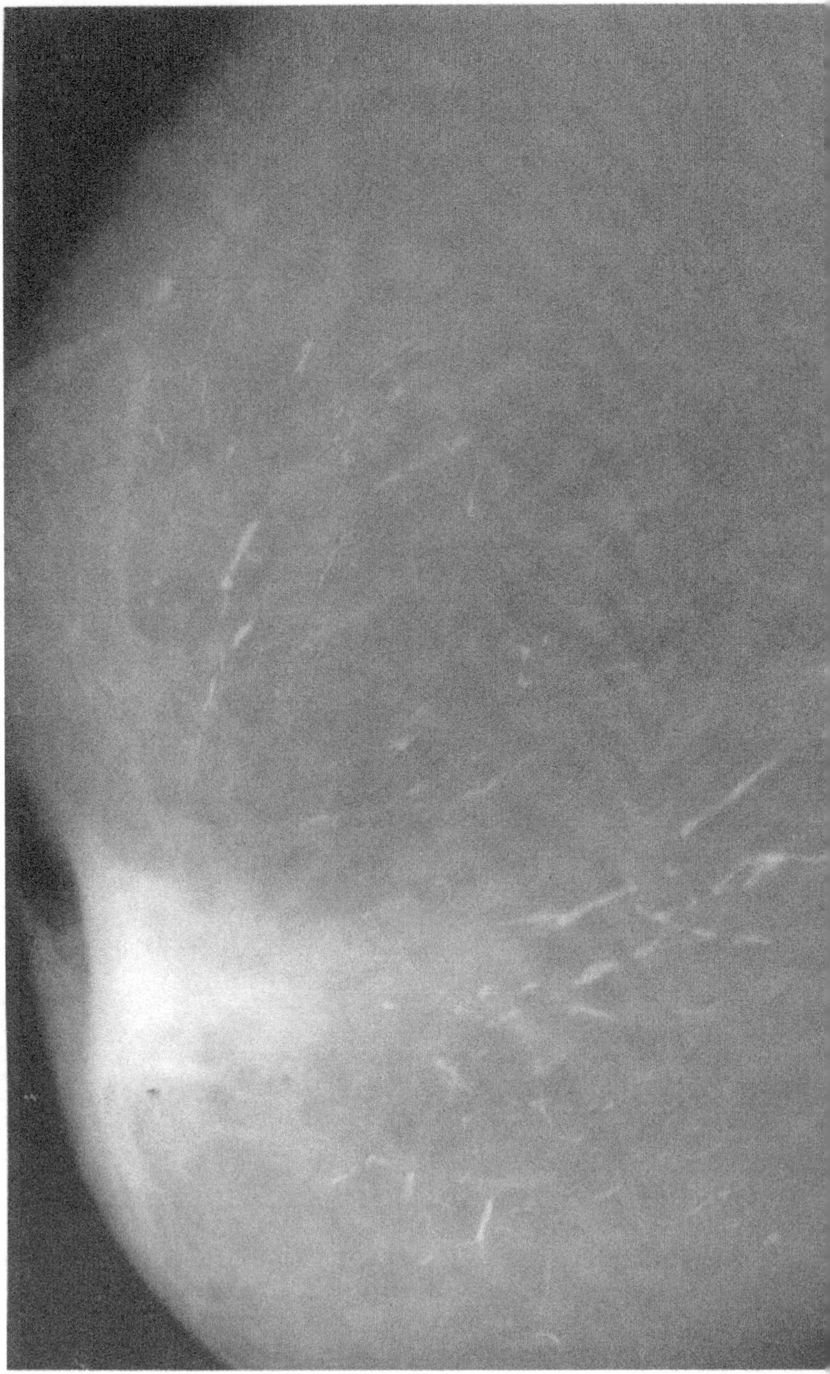

Postmenopausal woman with a history of severe pseudoinflammatory pain in **68** both breasts. Radiological investigation shows intraductal calcifications lining the ducts and their branchings.

This image corresponds to what most authors would call mastitis with plasmocytes, an inflammatory but abacterial condition occurring usually on ancient mammary duct ectasia. Histologically, it is a comedomastitis.

69

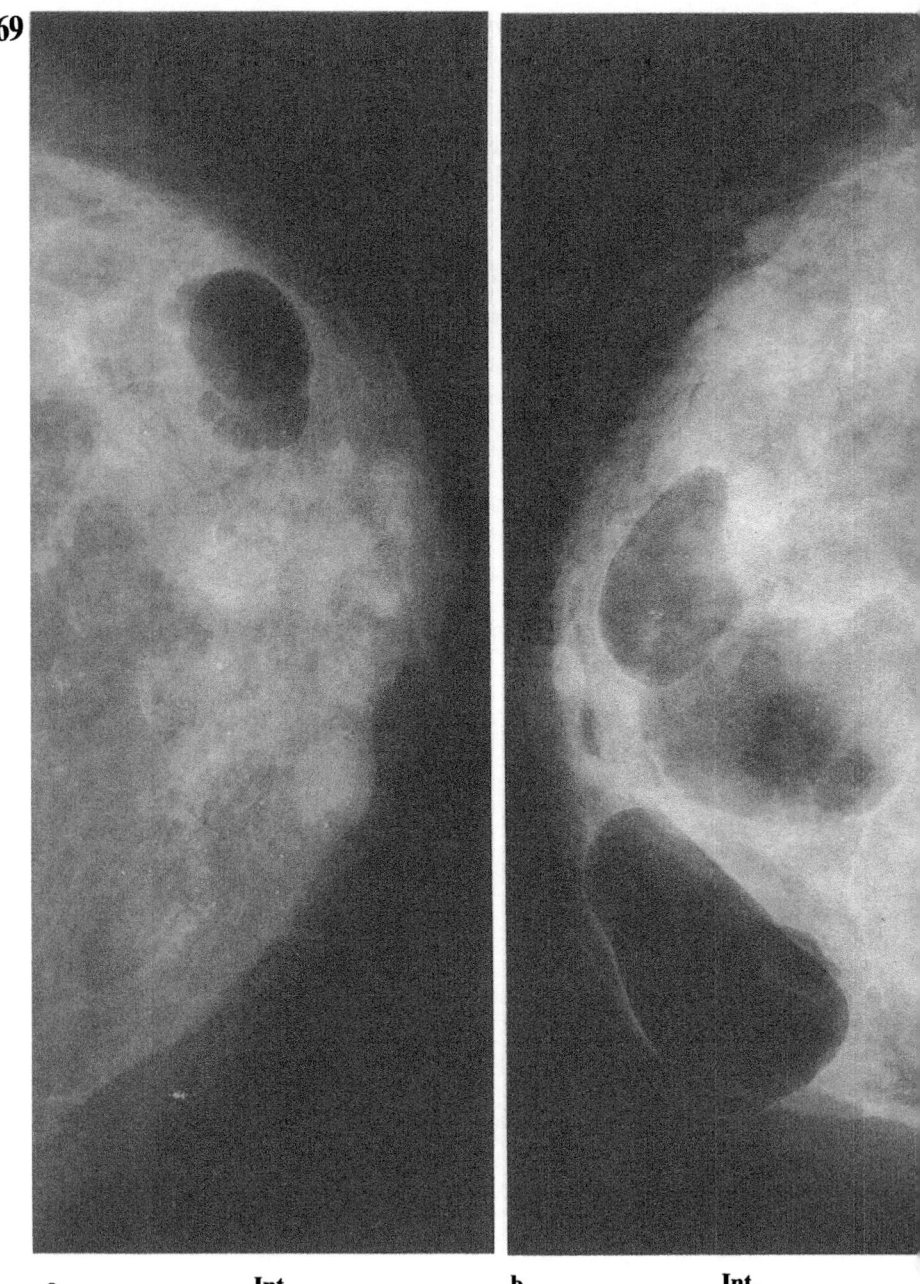

a   Int.   b   Int.

Puncture followed by air insufflation was performed in a patient with known and **69** followed-up cystic mastopathy.

The gaseous contrast permits visualization of bilateral calcifications (**a, b**); some are rounded, regular, and diffuse, while the others are finer and distributed in small clusters.

These two radiological signs associated with the presence of fibrocystic mastopathy suggest the diagnosis of lobular carcinoma in situ. Histology confirmed the diagnosis as bilateral lobular carcinoma in situ.

This case is a good example of the importance of cyst puncture followed by air insufflation. This procedure has not been superseded by ultrasonography since the latter fails to give evidence of calcifications, which are usually visualized in dense breasts only by means of the artificially created air contrast.

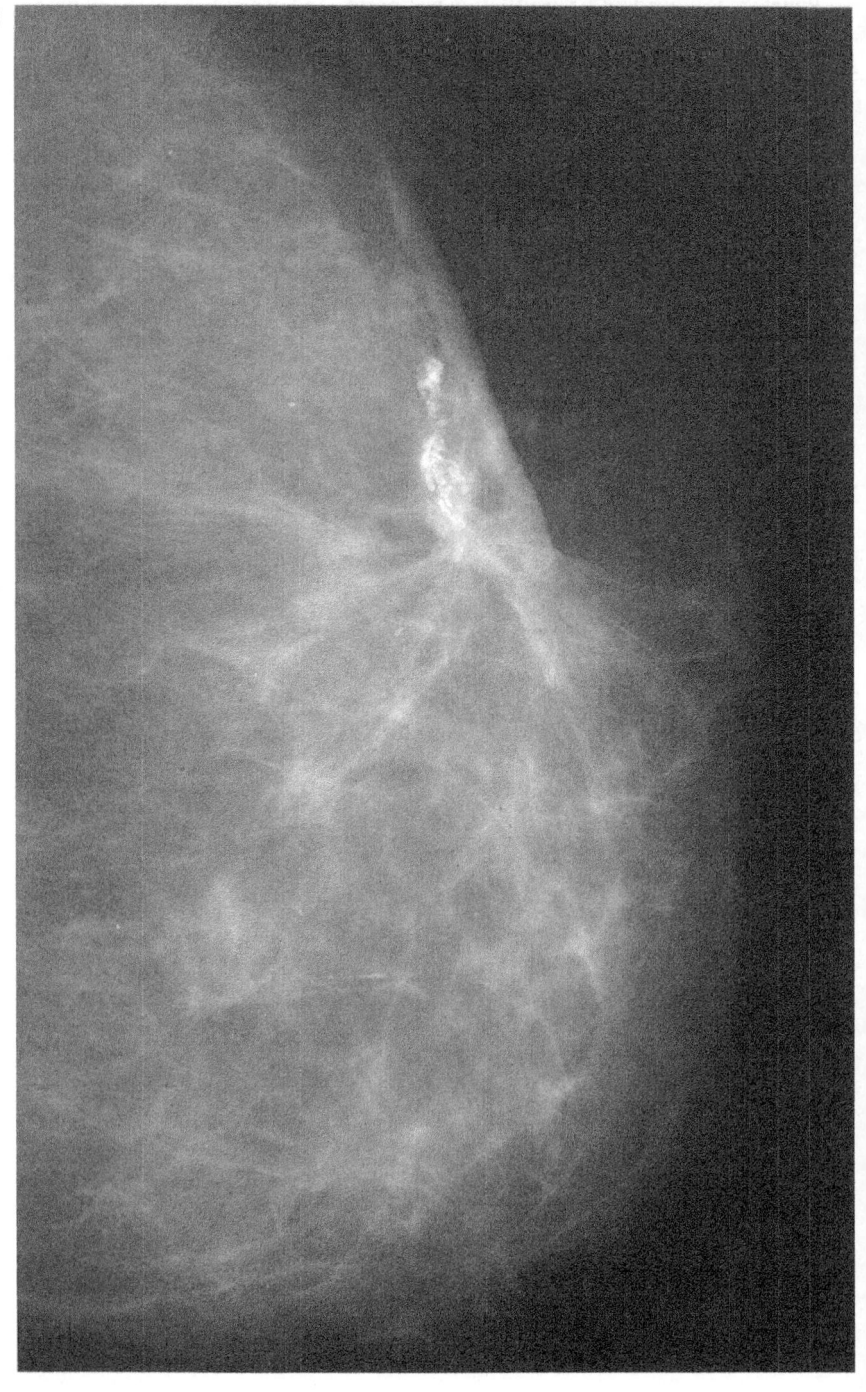

70

Image of a lateral scar with calcifications with clear centers of fat necrosis. **70**
Note the thickening of the fibrous bands, from the center towards the periphery, contrary to the stroma reaction surrounding carcinomas (appearance after radiotherapy).

71

a

b

c

Frontal (**a**) and lateral (**b**) views with spot film (**c**). These three radiographs show diffusion to the whole breast of typically malignant, highly polymorphous, dense calcifications arranged in clusters.

Although the histological examination did not give evidence of lymph node involvement, mammectomy was necessary because of the diffuse nature of the lesions.

These images correspond to what the histologists call intraductal diffuse comedocarcinoma.

72

a

118

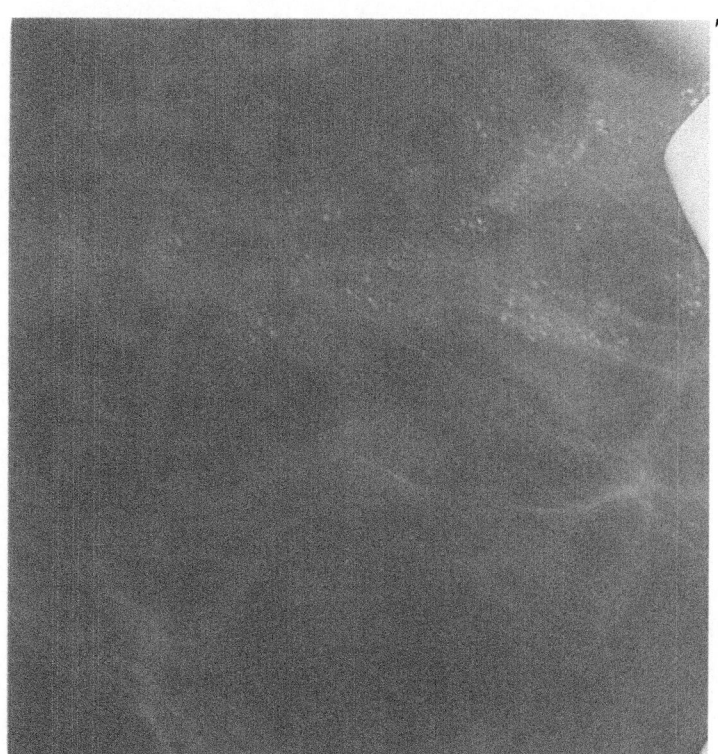

b

Detection of an intraductal carcinoma, recognizable by its calcifications, in a woman who came for a regular checkup (**a**). The spot film (**b**) permits very precise analysis of the polymorphism of these calcifications.

Histology showed a focus of microinvasion with metastases to the axillary lymph nodes.

73

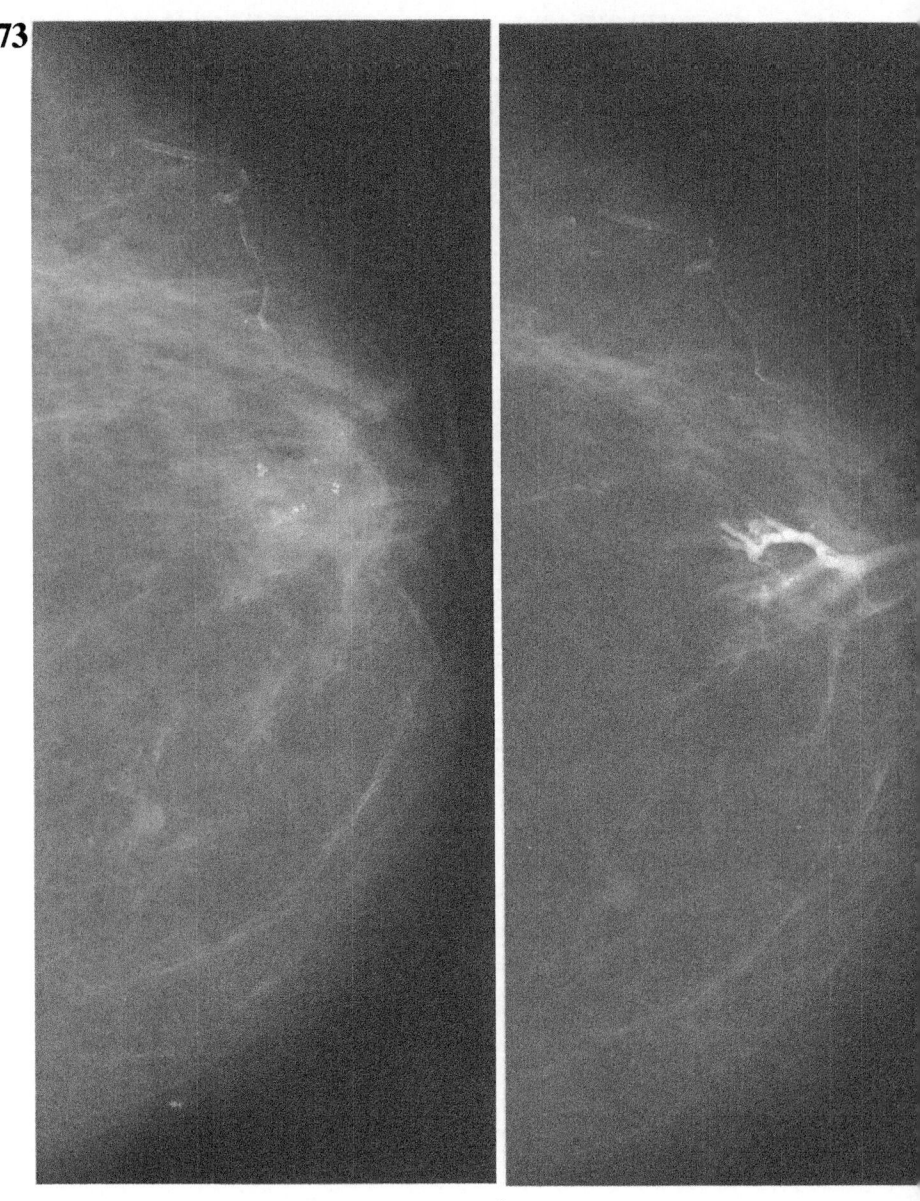

a   b

Radiographs made before and after galactography in a 71-year-old patient with
discharge of blood from the mamilla show the presence of highly heterogeneous
and polymorphous calcifications distributed in clusters.

Galactography demonstrates that the calcifications are strictly intraductal.
The plain film showed retroareolar linear opacities corresponding to lactiferous
duct dilatation due to discharge material.

Excision was performed and showed an intraductal plurifocal carcinoma.

VI. Intraductal and Intracystic Pathology

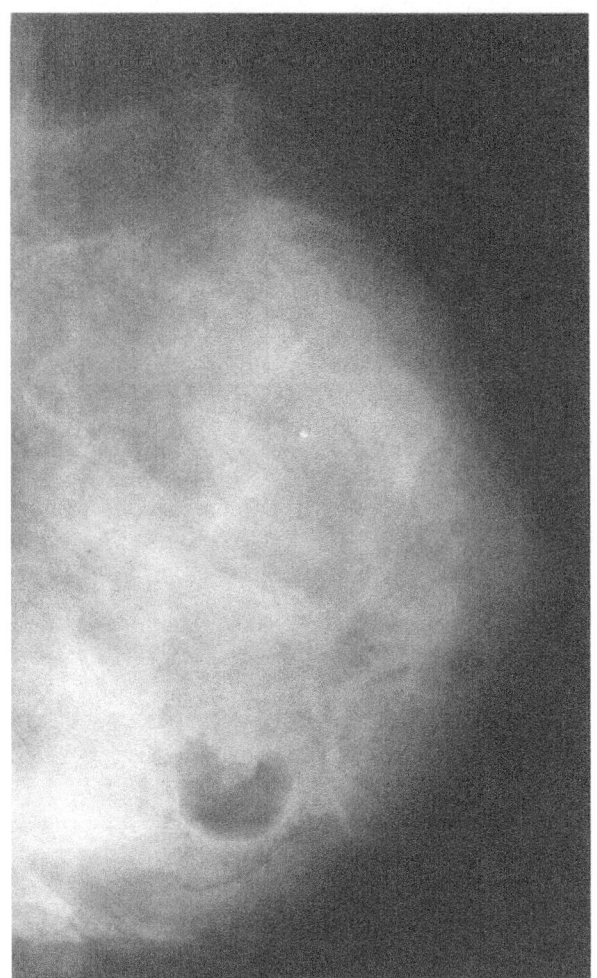

The film, taken after puncture of the cyst followed by air insufflation, shows relatively regular intracystic vegetation at the upper pole.

It must be kept in mind that there exists no radiological specificity sufficient to distinguish benign intracystic vegetations from cancerous vegetations; they often have the same mamillated appearance. Therefore, a cyst with vegetation must always be excised, whatever its radiological appearance after puncture.

In the case depicted, histology showed adenosis with atypical ductal hyperplasia.

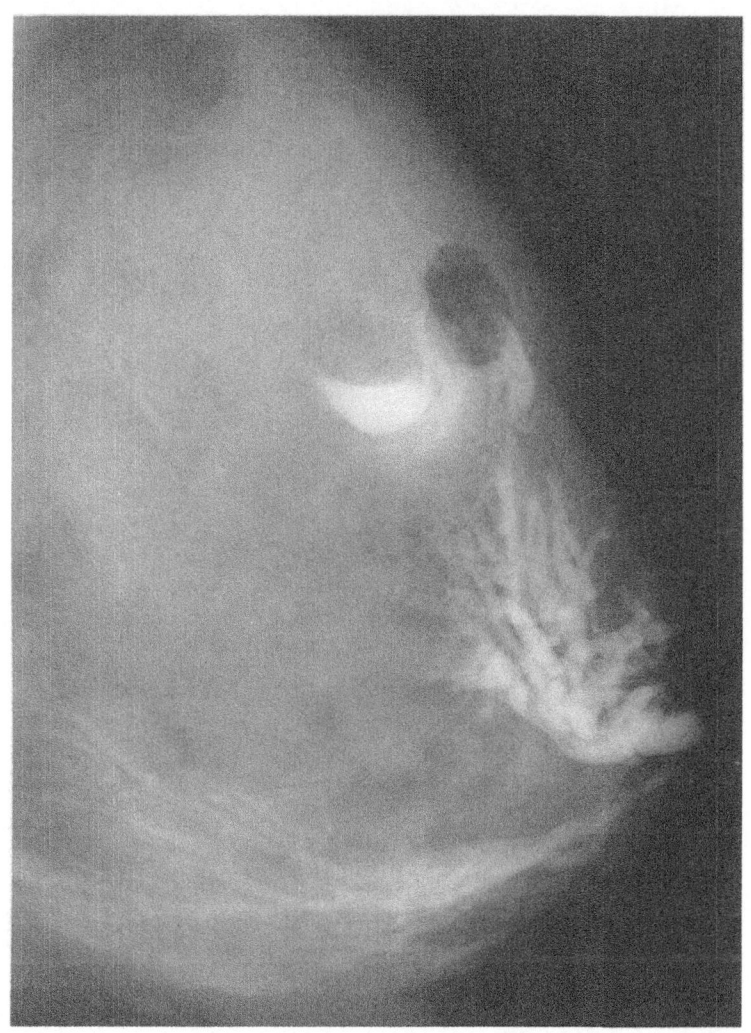

This radiograph, performed after puncture and air insufflation of two cysts and galactography, shows ductal ectasia and benign cysts, one of which is quite empty after insufflation; the other contains a significant amount of residual fluid which has been rendered opaque by the galactographic injection.

The radiograph is a very good illustration of the frequent coexistence of a fibrocystic disease and a secretory disease.

The two conditions are different entities, histologically and physiopathologically.

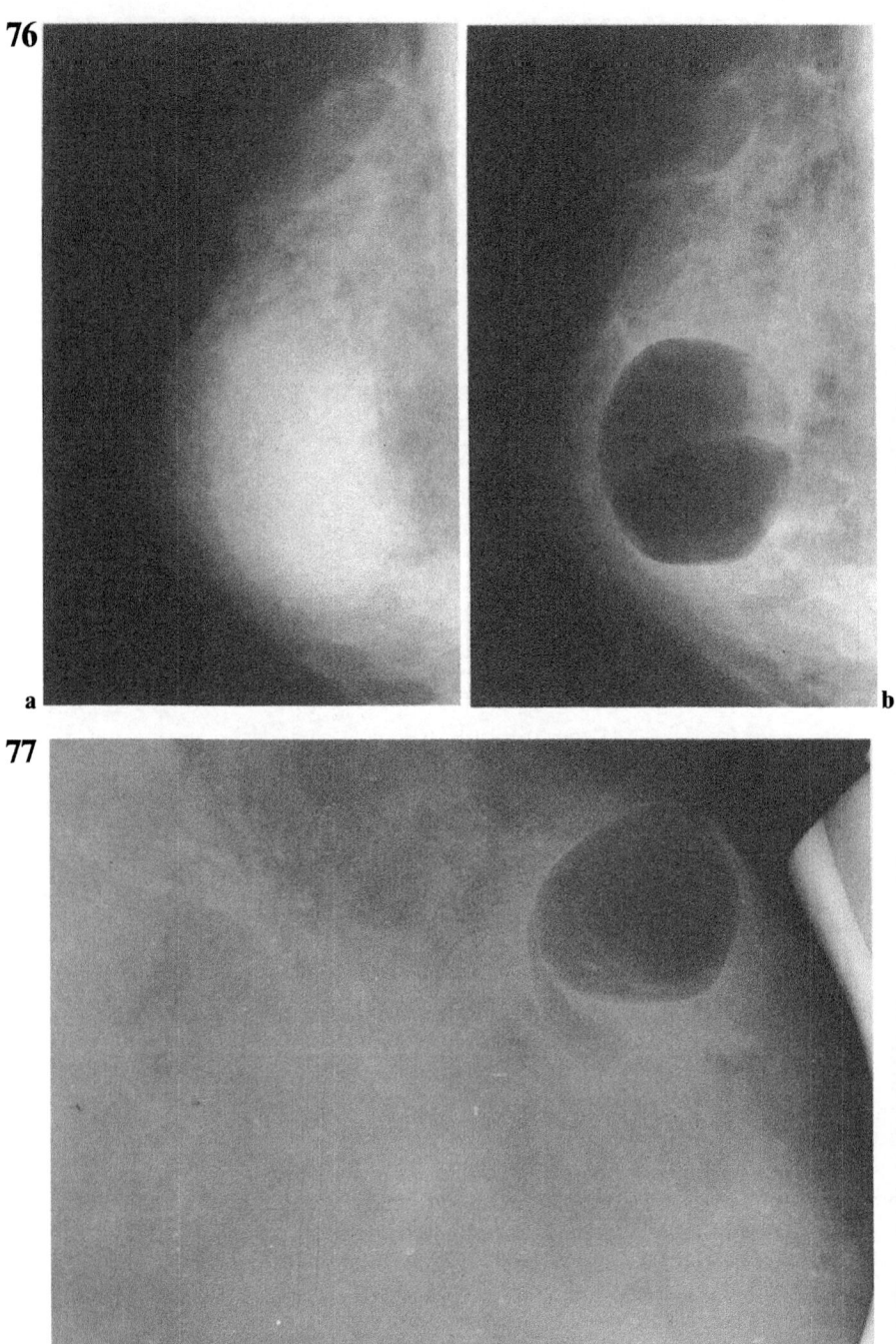

126

The lateral view, performed before needle aspiration (**a**), shows a dense, **76** homogeneous, rounded, and well-delineated opacity, integrated within a larger fibrotic patch, without signs of rupture in the structural organization.

After needle aspiration and air insufflation (**b**), the radiograph shows a quite benign cyst with a regular contour and an internal septation which had not been visualized on the film before puncture. No image of intracystic vegetations is seen.

Ultrasonography often reveals these internal septations.

This spot film perfectly demonstrates the importance of puncture followed by air **77** insufflation, which has not been supplanted by ultrasonography.

Through the transparency of the gas pouch created by the air insufflation one can faintly see numerous calcifications which would not have been visible in an opacity without insufflation.

In addition, these calcifications are diffusely distributed throughout the entire examined region. They are highly heterogeneous and polymorphous, and certain groups or clusters suggest the presence of a neoplastic lesion.

The histological investigation showed the presence of atypical lobular hypoplastic changes and of lobular in situ carcinoma.

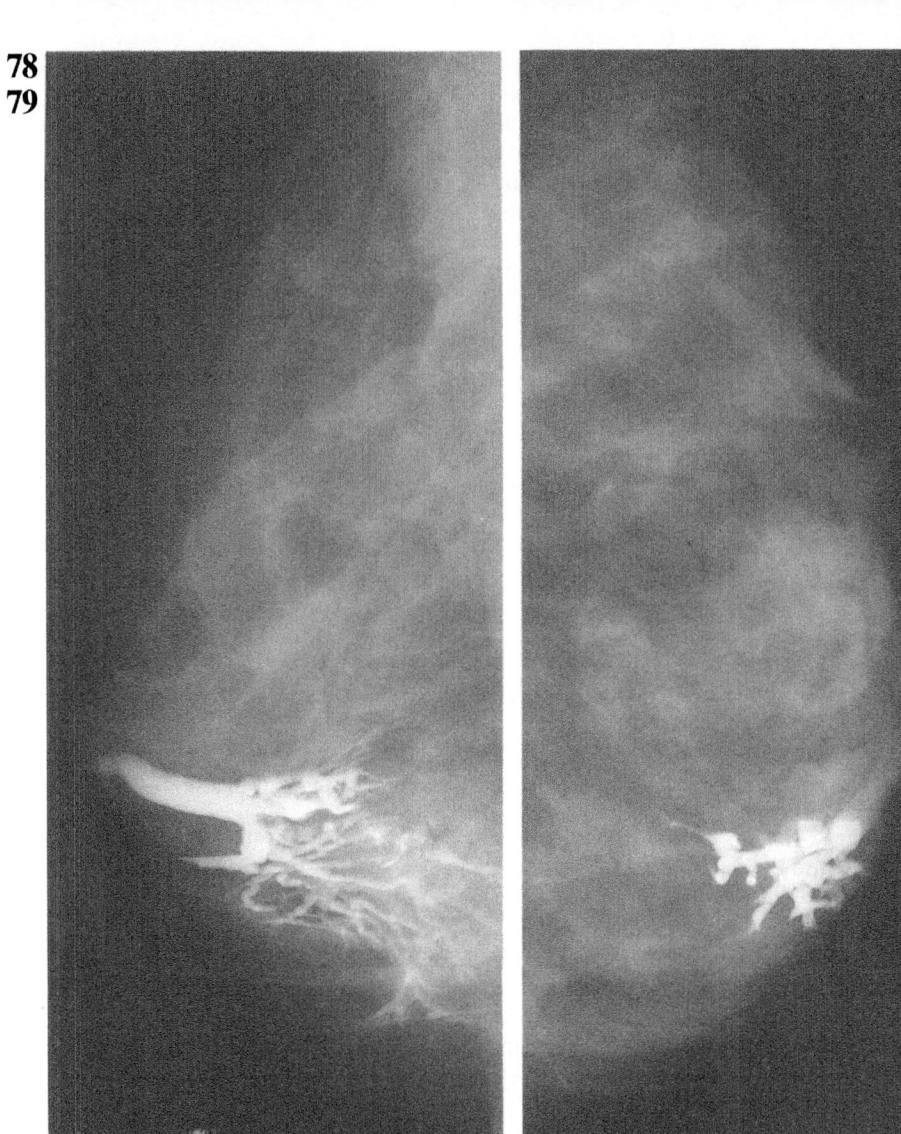

78
79

78   **79**

Injection of contrast medium into the lactiferous ducts reveals dilatation of the **78** ducts in the retroareolar region, as well as relatively tapered interruption of a duct in the infra-areolar region.

This image corresponds to diffuse canalar ectasia.

The radiograph performed before galactography shows a linear opacity in the **79** retroareolar region, which can be analyzed on the radiograph after galactography as canalar ectasia, spontaneously visible on a plain film.

Note that opacification is achieved only at 4 cm from the nipple due to partial obstruction of the lactiferous duct by secretion materials.

The histological diagnosis was ectasiating galactophoritis.

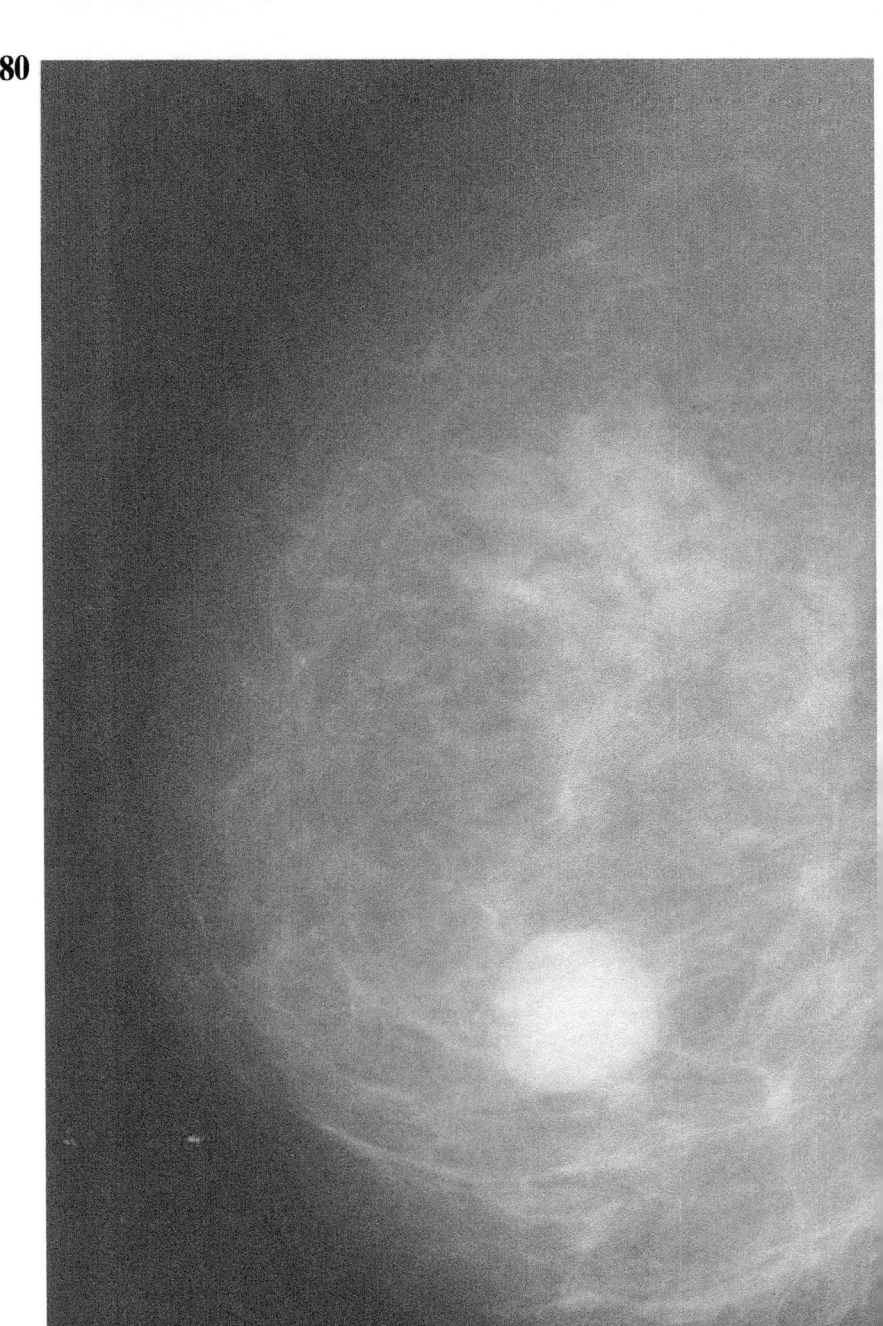

a

130

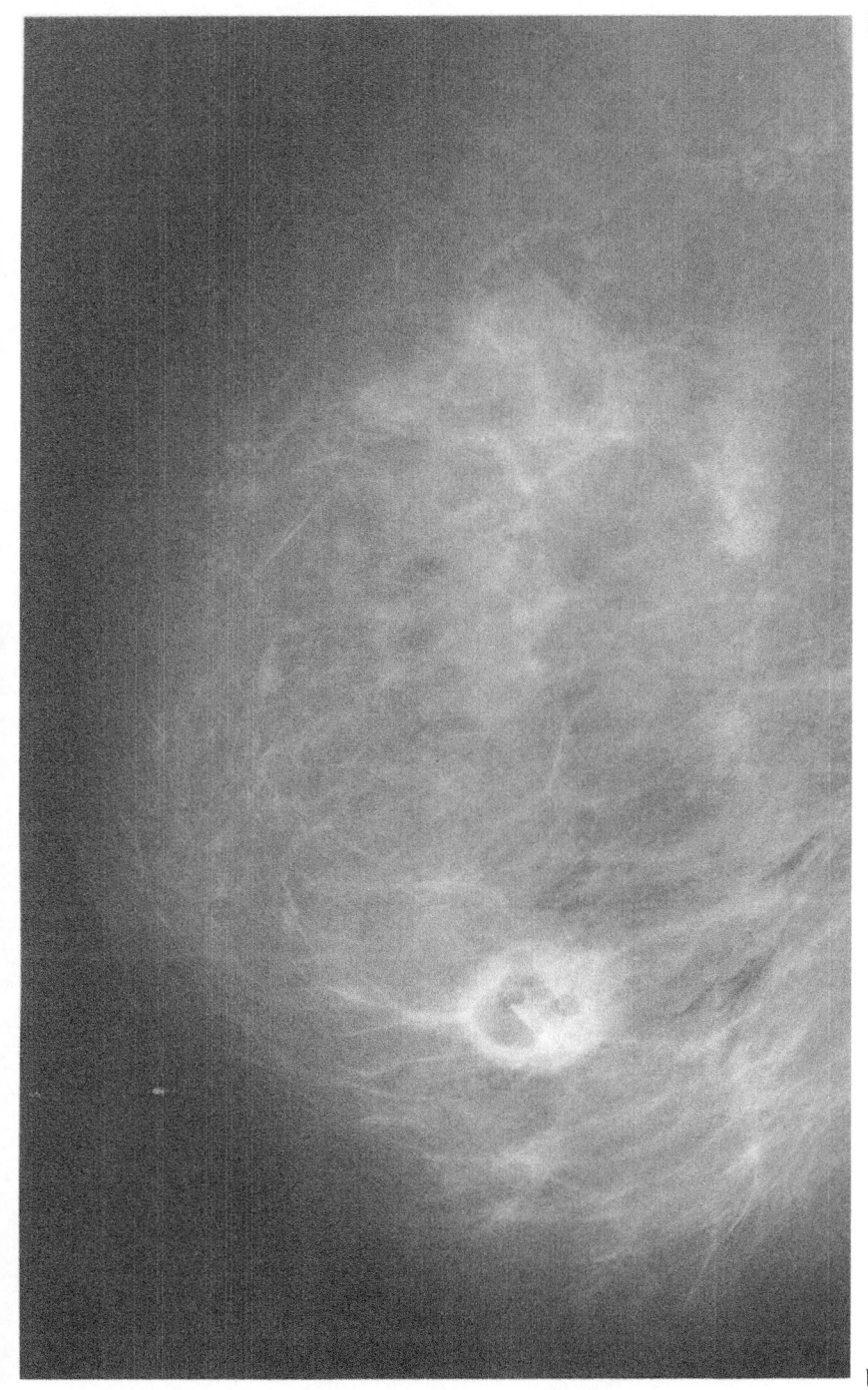

b

80

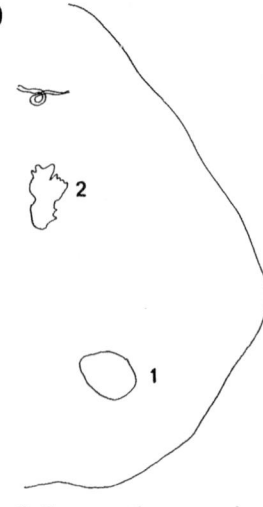

Films of the breast of a 56-year-old woman who complained of a nodule that had recently appeared in the left inferomedial quadrant.

The clinical examination indicated a benign cyst. Thermography revealed very marked hyperthermia overall.

On the radiograph performed before puncture (**a**), the nodule is seen as a dense, homogeneous, and well-delineated opacity, save, perhaps, for the anterior region, where the density is slightly uneven.

Important residual vegetation is seen after puncture and air insufflation (**b**). There is no radiological specificity and excision was decided on.

A close study of the radiograph reveals a relatively irregular, atypical opacity in the upper part of the lateral view, near the posterior margin; and some centimeters above, a dilated vascular loop.

1, Intracystic vegetation, i. e., an invasive papillary epithelioma; *2,* left superior nonpalpable scirrhous carcinoma.

81 Very good picture of galactography after contrast injection into several oozing pores, showing retroareolar ectasia of all ducts, but also the galactophorous system with appended small cysts.

This image demonstrates once more the frequent association of secretory and fibrocystic diseases.

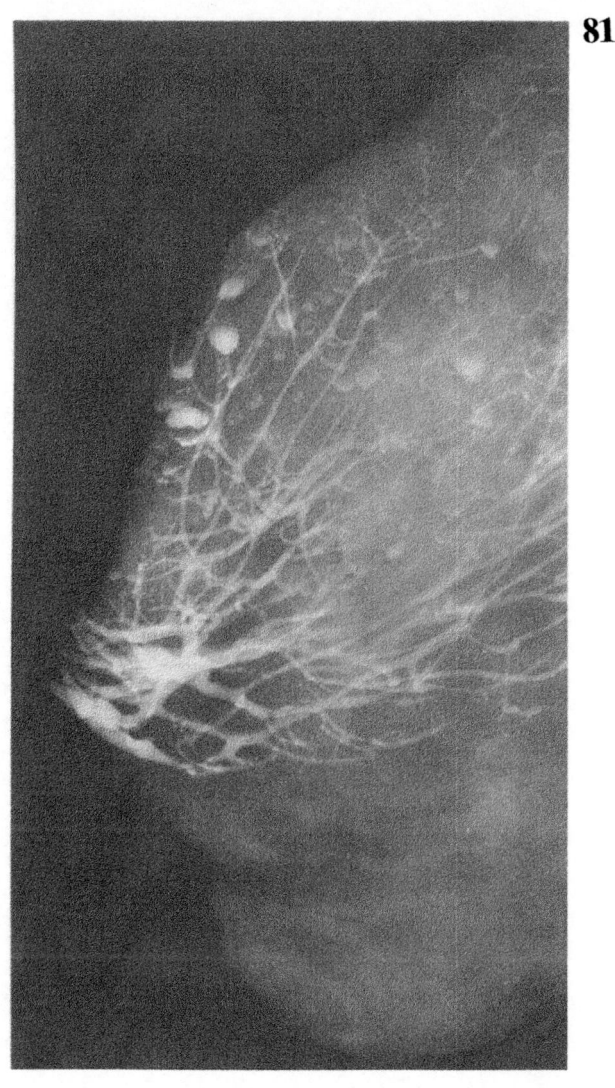

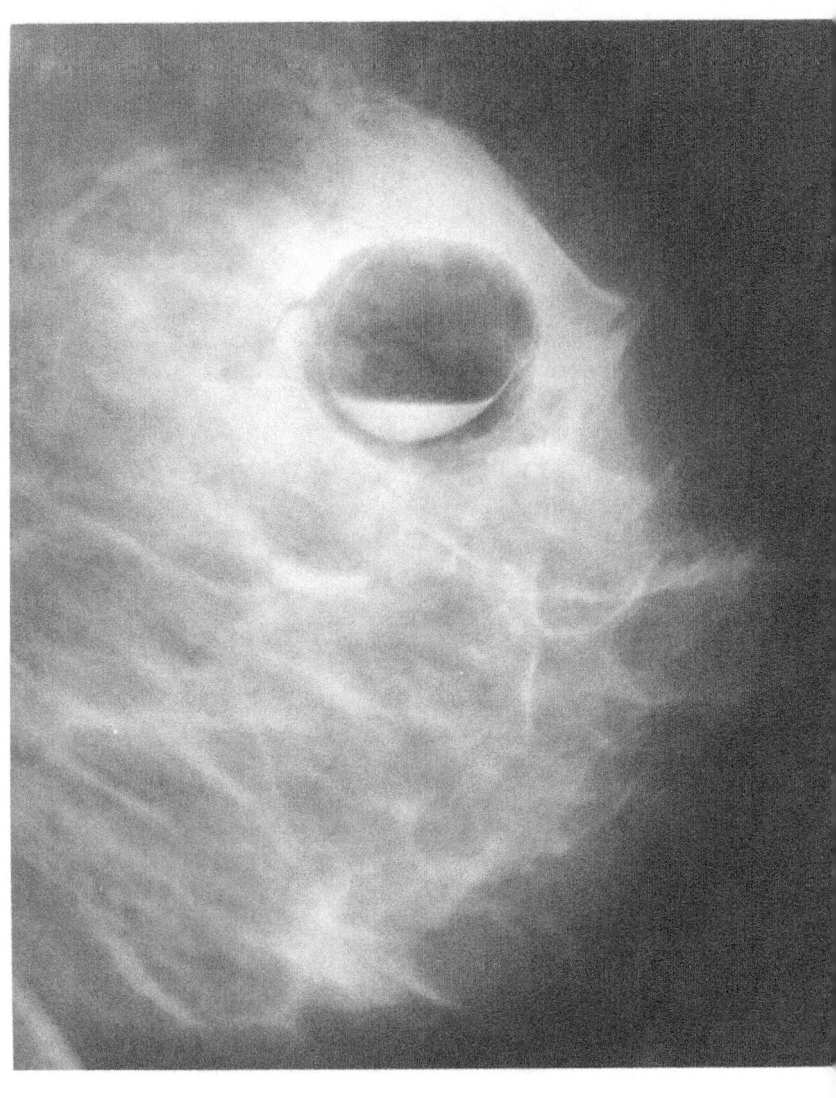

Example of a poorly punctured cyst with residual fluid in the lower part. Integrity of the lower part of the cyst cannot be affirmed, due to fluid superimposition.

In such cases it is advisable to perform a second puncture right away or a control after a short interval.

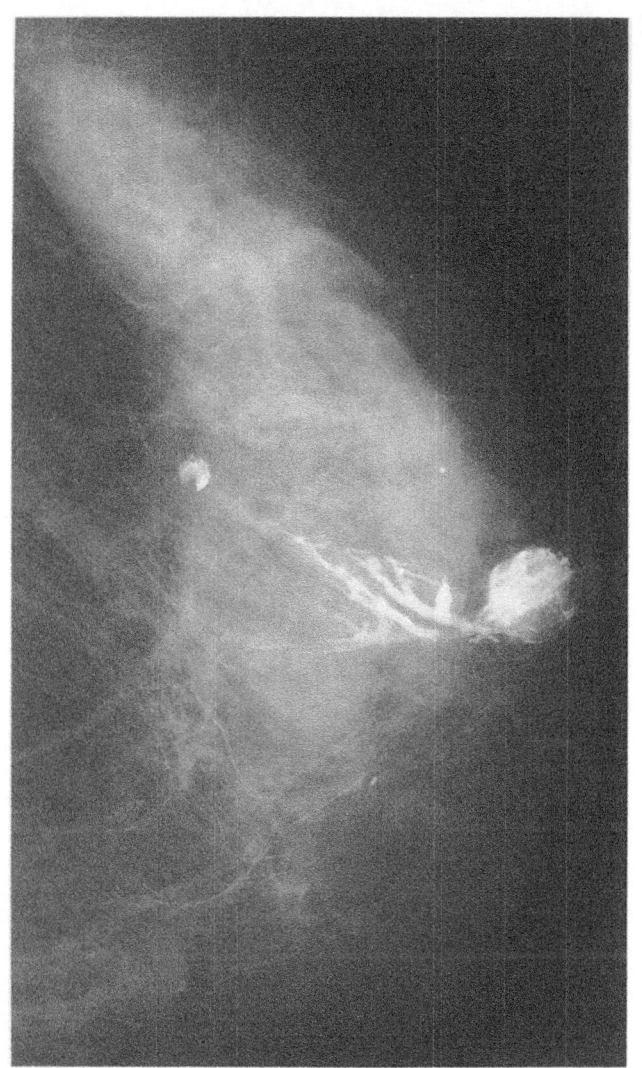

Galactographic examination showing retromamillary ductal ectasia and, in particular, a lacunar image in the dilated duct corresponding to a tumor.

No more than with intracystic pathology is it possible to ascertain the nature of intraductal opacities from the radiographic data. In any case, dilated ducts with intraductal vegetation must be dissected and operated on.

In the case shown here, the patient had a benign papillary tumor.

Subject Index